A CELEBRATION OF
SEX AFTER 50

DOUGLAS E. ROSENAU, ED.D.

JAMES K. CHILDERSTON, PH.D.

CAROLYN CHILDERSTON, M.A.

THOMAS NELSON
Since 1798

Published in Nashville, Tennessee, by Thomas Nelson. Thomas Nelson is a reg-
istered trademark of Thomas Nelson, Inc.

Scripture quotations noted NKJV are taken from THE NEW KING JAMES
VERSION. Copyright © 1979, 1980, 1982, Thomas Nelson, Inc., Publishers.

Scripture quotations noted NIV are taken from the HOLY BIBLE: NEW
INTERNATIONAL VERSION®, copyright © 1973, 1978, 1984 by the
International Bible Society, used by permission of Zondervan Publishing
House. All rights reserved.

Scripture quotations noted NCV are from *The Holy Bible, New Century Version,*
copyright © 1987, 1988, 1991 by W Publishing Group, a division of Thomas
Nelson, Inc. Used by permission.

Scripture quotations noted KJV are from THE KING JAMES VERSION of
the Bible.

Illustrations by Alan Tiegreen.

"I Am Woman" by Helen Reddy and Ray Burton. Copyright © 1971 Irving
Music, Inc. on behalf of itself and Buggerlugs Music Co. (BMI) All rights
reserved. Used by permission.

"You Are So Beautiful" by Billy Preston and Bruce Fisher. Copyright © 1973
Irving Music, Inc. and Alamo Music Corp. (BMI/ASCAP) All rights reserved.
Used by permission.

Library of Congress Cataloging-in-Publication Data
Rosenau, Douglas.
  A celebration of sex after 50 / Douglas E. Rosenau, James K. Childerston,
Carolyn Childerston.
      p. cm.
  Includes bibliographical references and index.
  ISBN 0-7852-6081-1 (pbk.)
  1. Sex—Religious aspects—Christianity. 2. Intimacy (Psychology)—
Religious aspects—Christianity. I. Title: Celebration of sex after fifty.
II. Childerston, Jim. III. Childerston, Carolyn. IV. Title.
  BT708.R635 2004
  306.7'084'6—dc22   2004002324

Printed in the United States of America

"Love is not love which alters
when it alteration finds"
—SHAKESPEARE

Lovingly dedicated to our parents
whose unaltered love we witnessed:

Carl and Doris Goltz – 58 years

Ward and LaVonne Childerston – 50 and counting

Eugene and Ernestine Rosenau – 55 years

Contents

Introduction

Maturity Rocks!:
Embracing New Truths About Aging

*Y*es, Baby Boomers, maturity does rock! This era of our fifties to our eighties represents an awesome time in our lives. We've paid our dues for wisdom and learned how to be comfortable in our own skin. We can create a higher quality of life—and pursue a fun, intimate companionship that may have eluded us in our younger years. Living life fully builds on the many tough lessons we have learned and is symbolized by our wrinkles and gray hair. We worked hard to earn these distinguished characteristics; wear them like medals of honor!

But somehow there's a disconnect. The truth is, most of us dread getting older. We would trade almost anything to be thirty or forty again. Why do many fear middle and old age, rather than embracing this wonderful stage of life?

Why do we chase youth and immaturity, and as a result lose the richness of this *capstone stage of the human life span?*

COMMON MISBELIEFS ABOUT AGING

The most obvious explanation centers in our false thinking about aging and our misunderstanding of what maturity means. We have bought into many myths that distort our attitudes and create dread or dissatisfaction. Here are some of the most toxic misbeliefs and the truths that dispute them:

1. Youth rules and old age stinks. We must maintain our youthfulness at all costs.

Truth: Like most things in life, a debit and credit column exists with positives and negatives during both youth and aging. Youth has more vitality and old age has more physical debilitation. Old age has a contemplative wisdom with the ability to slow down, while youth can be shortsighted and frantic.

Truth: Tight skin and firmer bodies may define youthfulness; but this does not equate to true beauty and sexiness as our youth-worshiping culture falsely thinks. Beauty is indeed in the eye of the beholder; wrinkles and softer bodies reflect a sign of maturity with its own sensuality. A constant striving for youthfulness can actually be immature and quite silly.

2. We can define the stages of middle- and older-age maturity using the same ideas and vocabulary with which we define younger stages.

Truth: This new phenomenon, higher levels of development, and greater skills of older years demand new vocabulary and concepts. An adolescent cannot be described with the concepts of infancy. What sixteen-year-old would want to be called cute and cuddly because he or she toddled around in such a precious way? Older age needs new lenses that extend beyond the way we would describe a thirty-year-old.

Truth: As will be developed in the rest of this introduction and book, old age presents new horizons and new levels of development and intimacy. Gray hair, years of living life, and maturity require a totally different way of looking at life and intimacy.

3. *Sexual desire and a longing for erotic connection are for the young and fade rapidly in our fifties and sixties.*

Truth: The body and hormones change, but couples can enjoy sexual interacting into their nineties. Sexual desire can stem from a caring and intimate relationship and has much more complexity than being totally hormonally based. Desire depends on the interaction of the body, soul, and spirit.

Truth: The lessons of maturity involve an ability to accept the imperfect, put a higher priority on companionship, and live in the moment. This can become a powerful catalyst for deeper sexual intimacy and meaningful lovemaking. True passion and enjoyable sexual connecting can increase with the empty-nest days and postmenopausal freedom.

4. *Great lovemaking depends on healthy, youthful bodies with stamina, flexibility, and exuberant intercourse and orgasms.*

Truth: Fulfilling lovemaking is about 20 percent physical and about 80 percent mental and emotional. Intimate sexual connecting involves much more than wild intercourse and explosive orgasms. "Playful, tender, trusting, and sensual" describe wonderful sex better than "intense, acrobatic, or all night."

Truth: It can be argued that to truly learn to *make love,* one must be at least fifty. Lovemaking involves a comfortable intimacy based on knowledge, acceptance, and tender eye-to-eye enjoyment of our lover. This grows with time together and a mature way of thinking and responding to life.

5. Pain and mishaps, which totally impede happiness and contentment, must be avoided at all costs.

Truth: The reality is that pain is a part of life and can be coped with graciously. We know that life, marriage, and love are complicated. Maturity can live with ambiguity and still experience joy and contentment. There's always plenty of ibuprofen, hot baths, and some contentment in the midst of pain and imperfection.

Truth: Many of the most important lessons grow out of experiences of physical or psychological pain and loss. The times of less pain become more enjoyable. Adapting to our limitations is a part of this adventure of aging.

6. Mortality should be feared, and aging bodies are a curse.

Truth: Understanding and accepting that we are in the last third of our lives makes every day more precious. We have different values, and quality of life becomes more crucial. The ability to slow down, relax, and enjoy recreation and relationships takes on special significance. Our aging bodies help create this important realization.

Truth: Mortality can be feared or embraced. Wisdom and maturity give us an ability to face this demon and gain a peaceful, godly understanding and acceptance. We are closer to death, but these deteriorating bodies are a sign our Creator is calling us home. This gives us new ways of looking at time, eternity, and the importance of relationships.

7. *Eternity and eternal values have little impact on this present life.*

Truth: We know our days are limited. A new realization occurs when we are faced with our mortality. These eighty-plus earth years are just a small part of our existence when we pair them with everlasting eternity.

Truth: God and the eternal values of living in His presence encourage us to build deeply intimate relationships. Maturity gives us new depth and perspective so that we can practice God's love (patient, kind, forgiving) in ways that will have eternal impact.

THE PARADIGM SHIFT FROM A YOUTHFUL OBSESSION TO A MODERN MATURITY

None of us can deny that dramatic changes occur in these mature years. The encouragement of this book is:

CHANGES bring **CHALLENGES,**
which present us with
CHOICES that can lead to
CREATIVE SOLUTIONS.

The part of aging that involves pain, deteriorating bodies, and facing our mortality isn't easy to work through.

We will never say that all of the changes should be cele-
brated. Aspects of aging are frustrating, but maturity can be
magnificent. Our deep belief is that the after-fifty years are
the best part of the life span. However, this requires an attitude that accepts challenges, choosing to turn them into
creations of intimacy and comfortable solutions.

Let's be fair, there are probably days with each of us
that we wonder if there are any solutions. The body has
sagged or we are having the menopause from hell or the
penis and orgasms just aren't the same. We are tempted
to take the low road:

                                                    Creative Solutions
                                                          ↗
Changes → Challenges → Choices
                                                          ↘
                                                    Negative Existence

But, pessimism and believing the myths can cause us
to grow increasingly bitter and resentful. We hope this
book will encourage and facilitate many of those positive and creative solutions. We need one another as we
support and fight our way through the difficult times
into hopeful solutions.

Many older people find that long-term relationships
have created a comfortable joy in their lives. We believe
it is a truism that "old dogs learn more tricks!" Maturity
has learned that it is insanity to keep doing things in the
same way and expect different results. We choose, sometimes reluctantly, to take challenges through to creative
solutions. The power of maturity can exist but be derailed

by myths and distorted thinking. Let's face it, we will have to dramatically shift our beliefs and attitudes to take advantage of our potential.

As we are confronted by the myths about middle and old age, a *paradigm shift* seems desperately needed. The idea of a "paradigm shift" conveys a wonderful variety of concepts. We're describing a complete shift in thinking and acting—so that we move outside the box and create *a whole new perspective* with a new vocabulary.

I [Doug] was at a party recently with friends in their fifties and sixties. I heard so many comments: "You look great—you're sure not showing your age." "He doesn't look a day over forty." "That haircut is so youthful." "She could put a thirty-year-old to shame." I felt like getting up on a chair and shouting, "People, we're in our mature years. Who cares about being described as being thirty years old?"

It made me aware that we need new attitudes and ways of appreciating one another: "Wow, your gray beard is distinguished." "You sure are spry." "What a wonderfully wise way of approaching your mother's nursing home." "I admire the courage you are showing in bringing Bill through his prostate cancer."

If we who are hitting our fifties and older will band together and embrace this paradigm shift, amazing results can occur. We can dispute our misbeliefs and develop a new and wise way of dealing with aging. It's been fun writing this book with the comradeship and fun humor of fellow older adults. (We've been asked if *A Celebration of Sex After 50* will be listed under fiction or nonfiction.) We understand one another, and our joking, though it seems like dark humor to someone in their thirties, gives us perspective on our aging bodies and changing values. Down deep we know:

Changes bring **challenges**, which present us with **choices** that can lead to **creative solutions.**

Maturity rocks. We think you will see this as the book progresses. Work on a whole new attitude about aging as you make a true "paradigm shift."

Chapter 1

Only Grown-ups Need Apply:
The Secret to Great Lovemaking

hat would a thirty-five-year-old say is the key to great lovemaking? Perhaps they would desire some powerful technique or to learn unique skills or develop a gymnast's body to make them stand out as a lover. Maturity knows better! These aren't prime bodies, and gymnastic moves aren't necessary. If there were a magic technique, we would already have discovered it. No, we know that lovemaking builds on who we are as a person and the intimate connection we have developed with our lover. The following formula sums it up:

Great Lovemaking = A Whole Grown-up Person + A Healthy Intimate Relationship

GREAT LOVEMAKING

Remember our insistence on shifting the paradigm as we create new attitudes? If we define "great lovemaking" as fantastic intercourse and wild orgasms based on an always-functioning body (penis and vagina), we are sunk. But that doesn't fit God's definition either. Go back to the beginning of time and think through why the Almighty created sex in the first place. God is Love, and humans are created in His very image to love. Nowhere is this more clearly revealed than through God's grand metaphor for intimacy—sexuality.

God created sexuality to reveal Himself and the value He places on intimate relating. He needed His human creation to understand what love is all about. "So God created man in His own image; in the image of God He created him; male and female He created them" (Gen. 1:27 NKJV). So marriage and great lovemaking foster intimacy and being "naked and unashamed." It transcends bodies, intercourse, and orgasms to the very soul of deep connection. How does this meaningful sex happen? Why can someone who is sixty better appreciate great lovemaking?

A WHOLE GROWN-UP PERSON

It's scary to realize that being a great lover depends on our personal maturity and growth. Neither our mate nor our chronological age can make us a grown-up. We are individually responsible for our character development and self-acceptance. In a critical manner, it takes two whole people to create a whole relationship. $\frac{1}{2} \times \frac{1}{2} = \frac{1}{4}$ of a truly intimate relationship. The following traits are indispensable in becoming an enjoyable, self-assured, grown-up lover.

Playful

Making love is certainly built on the foundation of play. I [Doug] am reminded of Christ's teaching that to truly experience the kingdom of God, we need to become like little children. An important part of being childlike is reveling in the awe of the moment and exhibiting uninhibited excitement and curiosity. Children are great teachers of amusement, as I learn every time my granddaughter and I hang out together. She squeals, claps her hands, and is awed by life. I've taken the liberty of paraphrasing Christ's advice in Matthew 18:3: Unless you become childlike and learn to be playful, you will never experience God's kingdom of unbelievable intimacy.

Learn from children's playfulness, which is perhaps best described by the terms *uninhibited excitement, eager curiosity, lighthearted fun*, and *spontaneous frolicking*. Kids can be self-directed and demand pleasure. In their childlike mentality, life is a big playground, and they expect to have fun. Playfulness is the ability to be unpretentious and candid as you demand things with enthusiasm and laughter—expecting your needs to be met.

Being childlike lends itself to aging and maturity. Who cares what others think as we try new behaviors? We've been disciplined too long—let's let loose and indulge curiosity. Time exists for more lighthearted and spontaneous fun. We know that playing has a way of connecting people. Gentle teasing, shared games, and mutual laughter can be bonding. Even sexual mistakes can create a playful memory. Life is too short to let false pride or inhibitions get in the way.

Time Out: Take time when you are out this week to stop and buy yourself a toy or two that would encourage you to play. You may want some that you and your mate can enjoy together, such as water pistols, rub-on tattoos, an edible lotion, or a board game.

Loving

An important part of love is respecting and unconditionally accepting your mate. If you want to find and focus on flaws, you will put a damper on your partner's attractiveness and the whole lovemaking process. Allowing your mind to become preoccupied with the natural body changes of aging can be very destructive. Your vocation as a mate is the nurturing and encouraging of your lover to revel in his or her sexual appeal.

Build some new attitudes. Remember that it is your lover you are enjoying and have become so comfortable with—that is what looking through the eyes of love is all about. Tender looks of shared history, a playful comfortableness, a growing eroticism that is based on intimacy and not firm bodies—yes, that is what love is all about. Again, your individual ability to love goes beyond your mate and his or her body or attitudes.

Don't assume that years together mean deeper love. You may need to forgive some old hurts and allow your mate to mellow in older age. A great love life depends on allowing your partner to apologize and change. We all do dumb things that can damage our lovemaking, and we need to be able to let go and move on. Mature love incorporates loving gestures that are nonsexual as well as sexual. Partners who are over fifty can place a special value on the hugs and caresses outside the bedroom that build a loving ambience and lay the groundwork for romance.

Time Out: While you are making love this week and enjoying each other physically, what are your mate's eyes conveying nonverbally? "I'm blessed to have you, thank you for all you have shared with me over the years." "I love the person you have become with your magnificent maturity."

Knowledgeable

It takes more than chronological years to become a wise and knowledgeable lover. First, become a student of your mate and yourself. The apostle Peter tells husbands: "Be considerate as you live with your wives" (1 Peter 3:7 NIV). An integral aspect of true consideration is constantly trying to better know and understand your partner. Your lover often knows what makes them smile or truly feel loved; do you? Meaningful lovemaking stems from this foundation of being happy and fulfilled together.

In the language of the King James Version of the

Bible, the word *know* is used to describe intercourse. For example, Isaac knew his wife, Rebekah, and they conceived a son. I used to think this wording indicated a reluctance of that culture to speak about or deal with sex openly. Now, I like this word *know* in our era of casual sexual encounters. Lovemaking should be "knowing" what your mate enjoys and needs. This knowledge takes time, curiosity, a good memory, and the willingness to be a student.

Time Out: Take a minute to do a quick personal inventory. Which areas of your sex life can benefit from greater knowledge? How are you going to implement change?

Clients will come to us believing something is very wrong with their bodily reactions and sex lives, only to discover that they are simply experiencing normal changes with aging. Study your mate's responses to know what is most enjoyable. No book can give you that information. Women, even more than men, vary about what feels good—the strokes and rhythms that are most pleasurable. This, of course, will change even more as we age. Be an eternal student of your partner's body and responses. Acquire a reservoir of knowledge of what excites your partner physically and mentally. Set the romantic mood, practice the right moves, and reap the exciting benefits of being a wise lover.

Honest

In making love, dishonesty destroys trust, fosters avoidance, and can create confusion and hostility. It may take the form of the dishonest husband who needs more physical stimulation to achieve arousal but is afraid to ask and avoids sexual interaction. A wife may be irritated by some touch that used to feel good or be struggling with loss of sexual desire during menopause. Rather than speaking up, she begins to resent her husband and his approaches—and his continued enjoyment of lovemaking. Both may also be unaware of their changing sexual needs and feelings—a more subtle form of dishonesty. It is not easy to be self-aware and truly transparent with our needs and feelings. It takes real maturity to openly discuss issues and confront changes.

Time Out: Do you have any dishonest sexual games you need to eliminate from your sex life? Do you hint or avoid, rather than talk through your needs? Have you asked your mate what he or she needs? Do you fear confrontation and settle for mediocrity? When your needs are satisfied, do you know this and feel fulfilled? Over the next week, take a half hour to discuss any dishonesty that has crept into your lovemaking.

Before leaving the character trait of honesty, let's acknowledge the ultimate kiss of death to a great sex life:

the extramarital affair. Sometimes in our fifties or sixties we wonder if we are still sexually attractive. Nothing can sabotage trust and the sacredness of a love life more than adultery. Sneaking, keeping secrets, broken promises, and divided loyalties rob a couple of sexual celebration in their marriage. An affair is a powerful negative illustration of the importance of honesty for sexual love to flourish.

Creatively Romantic

Grown-up lovers take the time to develop the sensual, romantic part of their minds and personalities. Every person has an exciting romantic side, but few take the time and energy to unleash their passionate capacities. Mates might be surprised at how talented and creative they can be in planning sexual surprises for each other—yes, even husbands who may appear to be romantically challenged. They easily come up with exciting, unique ideas as they focus on the importance of sensuality and mood setting—anticipation builds, and fresh attitudes pervade the whole sexual scene.

This will be developed in Chapter 20, but we believe with conviction that we can choose to never stop learning. Aspects of maturity encourage creative romance: more time and flexibility, a comfortableness in risking new behaviors, and creating greater quality of life.

Couples enjoy expressing their romantic nature. This may include surprise gifts, foot and leg massages, verbal demonstrativeness, a bath together, or dinner with candlelight and soft glances. Of course, romantic lovemaking doesn't always involve new techniques and experiences. There are certain positions, ways of caressing, places, rhythms, restaurants, moods, and vocabulary that remain enjoyable favorites. You will breathe life and excitement into the material of this book as you develop your imagination, relationship, and character traits.

Time Out: How would you define *romantic?*: creating moods, remaining sensual, recapturing the mystery, enjoying spontaneous passion, promoting tender sentimentality? Many wives and husbands wish their spouses would be more romantic. Make a brief list of behaviors that you consider romantic and practice one or two this week.

Disciplined

Discipline may seem an odd character trait to include for a fantastic lover. Most people think of discipline as the opposite of spontaneity, playfulness, and creativity. The truth is that an undisciplined lifestyle will end up producing very infrequent and disappointing sex. In fact, the creation of a scheduled time for sex will allow you and your spouse to anticipate and plan for creative and playful intimacy, with the possible added benefit of increased arousal. Discipline doesn't have to destroy the fun and spontaneity of sex or put pressure on you. The truth is that if you don't plan sex into your schedules and take advantage of *optimal* times, you will never make love with any frequency! The ambience, activity, place, timing, and technique are up to your romantic creativity. Just keep times sacredly reserved for sex.

Time Out: Put your heads together and plan when and how often you are going to make love each week as you allow time for love-making in your intimate companionship.

You have the promise of being a great grown-up lover. Incorporate the character traits of being loving, honest, playful, forgiving, knowledgeable, and disciplined. Practice these skills and remember, the formula for great lovemaking takes a whole, mature person:

Great Lovemaking = A Whole Grown-up Person + A Healthy Intimate Relationship

A HEALTHY INTIMATE RELATIONSHIP

Most people over fifty have figured out this crucial piece of information: *Having sex* and *making love* are two very different acts. Exciting sex doesn't necessarily create intimacy—rather, long-term, satisfying lovemaking flows out of an emotionally close and comfortably intimate companionship. Even with this critical knowledge, falling deeper in love and staying emotionally close don't come easy. The following four concepts are crucial in building healthy intimacy as a foundation for great lovemaking.

1. Filling the Love Tank—Trying Smarter, Not Harder

In marriage each partner has a love tank or a love bank into which mates make deposits through strategic loving deeds or withdrawals through negative behaviors. Part of great sex builds on a full love tank and feeling emotionally close—having the things done for us that make us feel loved. Bottom line #1: Some activities score points and some don't! Bottom line #2: Living with someone a long time doesn't guarantee you know how to fill their love tank.

Though sadly ineffective, we often practice on our mate what makes us feel loved or sexually aroused, hoping it will turn him or her on too. If your mate loves quality time spent together, a few candles or a quick back rub won't get the job done. What can be even tougher in this fifty-plus era of life is that some things that used to score points, like taking the kids for the afternoon or a quickie before work, won't work anymore and need to be revised.

Do you really want great lovemaking? Build real intimacy and remember, *it isn't how hard you try but if you are wisely pushing the right buttons.* Mature lovers learn what their mate enjoys and then remember and incorporate those things. If he speaks German, you learn a little German. If her language is French, you learn some French, no matter how difficult it is or how little sense it makes to you. When we are understood and our needs strategically attended to, we feel more in love and erotically inclined.

2. Affectionate Touch

Great romance and intimate lovemaking don't begin with sex. Feeling warmly attached through trust, tenderness, and *touch* produces the momentum. Remember the old adage that "embers reignite when placed in close proximity"? Similarly, emotional and physical warmth with tender emotions reignite physical closeness with your lover. "Feeling in love" and enjoying "gourmet" sex mean learning to *keep your hands and body in close proximity* to your mate. Find routines like cuddling before you go to sleep or going over and touching your mate whenever you walk by him or her.

3. Thoughtfulness, Surprises, and Tender Connecting

Thoughtfulness and choosing to be nice spill over into wanting to connect sexually. It's not much fun sleeping with the enemy or making love with someone who takes you for granted. Surprises, in a fun way, tell your mate that you thought of them when you weren't with them. It truly isn't the cost but the attentiveness and time invested that score points. Remembering to buy a small gift (that special lotion in her favorite scent) contributes to her feeling loved. Romantic sexual surprises are meaningful too. These creative innovations say to your sweetheart, "I thought of you and your pleasure. I'm stretching to reach out beyond myself to nurture you." For example, knowing her husband's continued enjoyment of her breasts, his wife bought lingerie just for his enjoyment.

4. Three-Dimensional Intimacy

Falling deeper in love and experiencing moving sexual intimacy demands that lovers bring body, soul, and spirit together. In the Garden of Eden, these three parts (of God's image in us) were comfortably joined. In an exciting way, this becomes one of the critical tasks in celebrating sex after fifty and shifting our paradigm to truly making love: learning to make love with our souls and spirits as well as our bodies.

Time Out: Plan a surprise for your mate that will convey, "I love you and I thought deeply about what could bring a smile to your face."

Great Lovemaking = A Whole Grown-up Person + A Healthy Intimate Relationship

How wonderful to know we are old and wise enough to understand this important formula. Great lovemaking certainly is achievable as we learn to be mature persons with effective intimacy skills.

Chapter 2

From God's Love Manual:
A Biblical Celebration

Scripture has several examples of celebrating sex after age fifty. Abraham and Sarah not only had sex in their nineties, but actually conceived Isaac. (We're sure you are ecstatic that God hasn't chosen to duplicate such a miraculous conception in your golden years.) Luke 1 says the parents of John the Baptist, Elizabeth and Zechariah, were "very old" when she conceived. And if you're looking for inspiration, Noah was over five hundred years old when he fathered his sons. The Bible contains wonderful concepts that can enhance lovemaking at any age.

GOD'S IMAGE AND THREE-DIMENSIONAL SEXUALITY

Genesis 1:27 states, "God created man in His own image; in the image of God He created him; male and female He created them" (NKJV). Wow! God's image is reflected in both masculinity and femininity and the way these aspects interface and are attracted to each other. Gender and sexuality give us insights into the Almighty. He values differences and similarities within a complementary partnership, excitement and nurturing, procreation and recreation. Bottom line: God wanted to reveal Himself by placing a priority on intimate loving relationships, so He created man and woman and sexuality.

In further developing His metaphor of sexual intimacy, the Almighty gave man and woman three dimensions to their sexuality: body, soul, and spirit. The apostle Paul, seeing the importance of this concept, prays, "May God himself, the God of peace, make you pure . . . May your whole self—spirit, soul, and body—be kept safe and without fault" (1 Thess. 5:23 NCV). These three parts of our selves are interwoven dimensions. In making the paradigm shift in these mature years, it is important to balance the soul, spirit, and bodily facets of lovemaking.

These dimensions join together to create sexuality and intimate relationships. Our bodies beautifully combine hormones, blood vessels, nerves, and skin to create attraction and desire. Our souls involve our minds and imaginations, wills and choices, and hearts and emotions.

Our spirits give us true love and create the ability to become "one flesh" (see Gen. 2:24).

The apostle Paul deals with the fuller meaning of sexual interaction and intercourse as he talks about the temple prostitutes in the pagan worship of Aphrodite (1 Cor. 6:9–20). Some of the Corinthian Christians were getting sexual excitement and release by visiting the temple prostitutes. He writes, "Foods for the stomach and the stomach for foods ... The body is not for sexual immorality but for the Lord ... Do you not know that he who is joined to a harlot is one body with her? For 'the two,' He says, 'shall become one flesh.' ... Do you not know that your body is the temple of the Holy Spirit?" (vv. 13, 16, 19 NKJV). Paul emphasizes that sexual union has an emotional and a spiritual dimension; it is not like eating a meal or casually satisfying a bodily desire. Sexuality is truly three-dimensional, with body, soul, and spirit.

Without this three-dimensional companionship, sex becomes another buzz or fix that loses its perspective and has increasingly diminishing returns. Going on a roller coaster or eating a big steak is fun, but we wouldn't want to do that two or three times a week the rest of our lives. Marriage to our soul mate—that is, the *spiritual, mental, and emotional* merger of wife and husband—allows sex to be ever new and exciting. Sex is a means to an end and never an end in itself. Making love unites and excites, but the relationship gives the context and meaning. Without true three-dimensional lovemaking, we find that sex becomes an activity (like eating steak or shooting white-water rapids) that quickly loses its dynamic appeal.

Time Out: 1. Sit across from each other nude and gently place a hand over each other's heart. In the quiet, feel life pulsing in the body of the one you love. Close your eyes and sense the closeness that is being allowed by a person that needs and loves you.

2. Look deeply into the window of the soul, the eyes, and communicate love with no words spoken. Eye-to-eye sex is special, and it doesn't have to include constant eye contact.

3. Write down and practice some of these affirmation statements: "When I hug you for a minute or more, the world disappears," "I don't know why you adore me, but I am glad God gave me to you," "When you are inside me and hold me tight, I feel we blend into a oneness I can only feel but not describe." Okay, so you may need your own words, but say them out loud.

THE MARITAL UNION

God stated in the beginning of creation, "It is not good that man should be alone; I will make him a helper comparable to him" (Gen. 2:18 NKJV). Not only did God create the genders, He also designed a special, unique mating relationship: "The Scripture says, 'So a man will leave his father and mother and be united with his wife, and the two will become one body.' That secret is very important—I am talking about Christ and the church" (Eph. 5:31–32 NCV). "The man and his wife were naked, but they were not ashamed" (Gen. 2:25 NCV). Making love and creating a one-body partnership are a profound, mysterious, and dynamic process.

As mature lovers, we realize something is lost if we treat making love as simply physical excitement, intercourse, and techniques. Making love offers insight into Christ's relationship with the church. It includes joy, excitement, trust, commitment, unselfish nurturing, self-esteem, and a mutually fulfilling, comfortable, playful companionship. We will never completely comprehend this "secret" of intimacy or, as some scriptural translations state, this "profound mystery."

It is tremendously moving to think of God's original one-body companionship. Adam and Eve, before the Fall, had the marvelous capacity of being totally naked, physically and emotionally, with no shame or fear. They reveled in a childlike trust and curiosity—laughing, exploring, giving and receiving love. Sex was a glorious, innocent celebration lived out with instinctual honesty, respect, and zest for life.

First Corinthians 7:3, 5 tells about the importance of staying sexually connected in marriage: "Let the husband render to his wife the affection due her, and likewise also the wife to her husband . . . Do not deprive one another except with consent for a time . . . and come together again so that Satan does not tempt you because of your lack of self-control" (NKJV). In a loving partnership, enjoying sexuality and connecting with a mate are gifts each brings to the other willingly—*not by demands or coercion.*

Please don't use God's loving guidelines as weapons on each other. Some husbands and wives club their mates with this passage and say things like, "If you don't have sex with me tonight, you are sinning." The real sin is theirs because they have never taken the time, loving-kindness, and energy to make changes needed to appeal to their mates romantically. Becoming one body has ceased to be the loving gift of meeting each other's needs and uniting. Making love is about giving—not demanding.

On the other hand, are you too fatigued or busy or inhibited to have sexual relations regularly? If so, you, too, are missing God's plan for marriage and the enjoyment of one of His avenues for increasing intimacy. Failing to structure frequent sexual activity into your companionship may open you to Satan's temptations. Please hear our heartfelt advice: Get counseling and do whatever God needs you to do to get sex back into your marriage! As we tell Christian couples, "A meaningful sex life in your marriage is one hill worth dying on. This is not optional in God's eyes."

There is no replacement for what God intended sex to do for intimate marriages. The Creator set no age limits. Lovemaking in our fifties or eighties continues to be the framework for expressing many powerful and exciting emotions. Making love also helps dissipate and defuse negative emotions and behaviors, like hostility, nit-picking, and defensive distancing. Spouses who frequently play together sexually stay together in a warm and bonded way, keeping at bay many of the dragons that can hurt intimate companionship.

Godly Submission Versus Self-Focus

Mature lovers need to be able to practice both submission and a righteous self-focus in the marital union. We as Christians are encouraged to be submissive. That is, we are encouraged to place our partners' needs and feelings ahead of our own. And submission is a significant part of a great sex life. Through submission, we honor our mates and nurture them unselfishly in ways they truly enjoy. We can give as gifts sexual favors that our mates desire, but may not be as important to us.

But fulfilling sex also requires being selfish. If we are always other-focused, and if we always repress or ignore our own needs, we forfeit complete sexual fulfillment. Intimate lovemaking is a partnership with both selfishness and unselfishness. Great lovers know their own bodies and enjoy their sexual feelings. This is part of the reason why some women become more sexual in their forties. They know more of what they want and enjoy and are more assertive in expressing this.

Self-focus doesn't seem to get equal time in practical Christian training. Self-awareness and taking personal responsibility are crucial to building a healthy sexuality. The Bible commands us to "love your neighbor as yourself" (Mark 12:31 NKJV), and it states that "husbands ought to love their own wives as their own bodies" (Eph. 5:28 NKJV). These teachings are based on the idea of a healthy self-concept.

As Christians, we are accountable to God for creating a good sexual self-image and accepting ourselves without comparing ourselves to others. We are answerable individually to build a vibrant self-awareness and to learn to love and appreciate our bodies' potential for sensuality. We need to understand our own sexual needs and assertively fulfill them.

Orgasms are an excellent example of healthy sexual selfishness. Your mate does not experience your orgasm. You focus on your sexual feelings and allow them to build to a climax. This is an intensely personal pleasure within your mind and body. You selfishly let your mind enjoy the intensity of your excitement and orgasm but unselfishly allow your mate to observe how much pleasure your mate brings to you. Your partner is aroused by your personal excitement and intense experiencing of erotic release. This self-focus creates a mutual intimacy that encourages bonding and can be a great aphrodisiac.

Time Out: Individually, make a list of three things you would like to do that could increase your personal enjoyment of love-making and three ways you could please your partner. Share this list with your mate and discuss. How has your list changed in these more mature years?

THE "WATER" OF INTIMACY

A wonderful scriptural passage for us sex therapists is Proverbs 5:15–19:

Drink water from your own cistern,
    running water from your own well.
Should your springs overflow in the streets,
    your streams of water in the public squares?
Let them be yours alone,
    never to be shared with strangers.
May your fountain be blessed,
    and may you rejoice in the wife of your youth.
A loving doe, a graceful deer—
    may her breasts satisfy you always,
    may you ever be captivated by her love. (NIV)

We could paraphrase this for wives:

Rejoice in the husband of your youth.
A gentle stag, a strong deer—
    may his hands and mouth satisfy you always,
    may you ever be captivated by his love.

The Bible often uses water as a powerful and fitting metaphor for cleansing, healing, and rejuvenating. There are beautiful images like "streams in the desert," "water of life," and "beside the still waters." What a tremendous portrayal of the dynamic nature of lovemaking to compare it to a cistern, a well, a stream, and a fountain of water. It is like a cool, refreshing drink from your own safe supply.

In one way, your marital sex life is like a cistern in which you have stored many amorous, erotic memories and a repertoire of arousing activities. You can dip into it again and again in your fantasy life for excitement and fun. In another way, making love is like a stream or spring of water. Sex in marriage has an ever-changing, renewing quality to it.

A routine sex life is not God's design, especially when maturity can help us learn new attitudes for enriching our intimacy. I appreciate the words *rejoice, satisfy,* and *captivated* in the Proverbs message. Pleasure and fun are an intended part of making love. It is important for mates to enjoy playing together. We can rejoice with the mate of our youth. Our creativity, imagination, and love allow us to remain enthralled with our lifetime lover.

An Erotic Celebration

Sex is an erotic celebration that only those over fifty can fully appreciate. As part of the paradigm shift, let us redefine the term *erotic* beyond the shallow Hollywood recreational concept of erotic that lacks depth or values. *Eros,* the Greek word for sexual love, includes the idea of fusion, passion, attraction, and bonding. Erotic love is getting lost in someone's eyes. Erotic love is mental imagery, anticipation, playfulness, ambience, and lovers physically enjoying each other. Song of Solomon contains many beautiful images of erotic love:

> Let him kiss me with the kisses of his mouth—
> For your love is better than wine. (1:2 NKJV)

> My lover is mine and I am his;
>   he browses among the lilies. (2:16 NIV)

> Your two breasts are like two fawns . . .
> Your plants are an orchard of pomegranates
>   with choice fruits . . .

You are a garden fountain,
a well of flowing water . . .
Let my lover come into his garden
and taste its choice fruits. (4:5, 13, 15–16 NIV)

My own vineyard is mine to give . . .
Thus I have become . . . like one bringing
contentment. (8:12, 10 NIV)

These passages so beautifully and poetically describe the erotic passion of three-dimensional lovemaking. Sex is the curious and excited exploration of each other's erogenous zones to create pleasure. We as lovers are to entrust our private parts to our mates, for, indeed, "my own vineyard is mine to give," and we should learn to have no shame or inhibitions with the genital area. We can create stimulating atmospheres, sharing choice fruit and drinking till contented from the flowing water of our sexual relationship.

Chapter 3

"Hear Me Roar!":
Female Sexual Changes

*A*s we approach the topic of female sexual changes that occur with aging, we're reminded of some lines of the Helen Reddy song that became somewhat of a feminist manifesto in the 1970s:

> I am woman, hear me roar
> In numbers too big to ignore . . .
> You can bend but never break me
> 'Cause it only serves to make me
> More determined to achieve my final goal
> Oh yes, I am wise
> But it's wisdom born of pain
> Yes, I've paid the price
> But look how much I've gained.

By the year 2030, 1.2 billion women in the world are expected to be age fifty or older. During the 1990s, approximately 24.5 million women worldwide reached menopause each year. In the U.S. and Canada alone, approximately 4,000 women reach menopause every day.[1] These numbers really are too big to ignore.

But what's the roar? That depends on the woman. Some women will respond with growth as they face the adversity of life, using the challenges presented by physical changes to gain the "wisdom born of pain" and develop a healthier new identity. For others the roar may represent their frustration, complaints, resentments, and losses as they unsuccessfully battle the aging process.

The key word that describes the shift in sexual function for women at midlife is *change*. A woman may experience her sexual desire subsiding or she may find desire increases. As a result, her frequency of sexual activity may increase or decrease. She may also experience an increase or a decrease in the sensitivity of her clitoris, and her sexual responsiveness may also go up or down. A wife may find that she experiences fewer orgasms and with unpredictable intensity, or she may realize an increase in orgasms and a sexual awakening.[2] It is impossible to foresee how an individual woman will experience midlife sexual changes, but we can predict that what was normal before may not be now. Many women will not experience a decrease in sexual desire during menopause, but when they do it is often due to hormonal imbalances, negative thinking, relational problems, or other stressors. The sexual changes in women may be less noticeable, but they are more variable and complex than the changes in men. This chapter will address female sexual changes that can occur from midlife onward, and in the next chapter we will focus more on the hormonal changes of menopause and how sexual response may be impacted accordingly.

PHYSICAL CHANGES

Thinning and Tightening of the Vaginal Wall

As levels of the sex steroids, estrogen and testosterone, begin to fluctuate, changes may first be noticed in the genitals. Dropping estrogen levels will cause the vaginal walls to thin, and they will not have the same elasticity and soft padding. The vagina may shrink, with its mouth becoming narrower.

Because the vagina has lost some of its cushioned effect, some women will experience urethritis (sometimes called the honeymoon disease, it is an irritation of the urethra and bladder from the penis hitting them during intercourse). The labia minora and labia majora (inner and outer vaginal lips) can also atrophy, thus leaving the clitoris more exposed. This means that direct stimulation of the clitoris can become painful.

Vaginal atrophy is a consequence of diminished estrogen production and/or lack of use. Many women have thus benefited from estrogen replacement therapy (ERT) and/or estrogen creams, which aid in restoring the vaginal wall and improving lubrication. It is possible to increase vaginal muscle tone by regular Kegel exercises, which involve pubococcygeus (PC) muscle contractions. These exercises are also very effective in maintaining vaginal blood circulation. Two hundred Kegels a day will go a long way in preserving the vaginal tissue by increasing blood flow to the area.[3] Adding more soy products to your diet is a natural way to boost estrogen, as soybeans contain phytoestrogens, which can rebuild and moisturize thinning vaginal walls.

Time Out: Here are two different types of exercises that you can practice to strengthen your PC muscle. They are easy to practice while in the car, on the telephone, or watching television.

1. Become familiar with your PC muscle (which goes from your pubic bone to your coccyx/tailbone and is the muscle you would contract to stop urinating) as you contract and immediately relax it. Do this rapidly five times as you inhale and then exhale. Repeat five times.

2. Pretend your husband's penis is at the mouth of your vagina and you are trying to suck it into your vagina by pulling with your PC muscle. Pull for three seconds and relax. Repeat ten times and then rest.

Decrease in Vaginal Lubrication

The loss of estrogen can affect lubrication too. It may take longer to lubricate, and the amount may be less. While in the past it may have taken seconds to create arousal and sufficient lubrication, it may now require several minutes of love play (for some women, dryness will require artificial lubrication). Vaginal dryness can be helped by regular Kegel muscle exercises in that as you increase blood circulation, natural lubrication will be enhanced. There are a variety of lubricants that can be used during intercourse to reduce irritation and friction. Begin by trying water-based lubricants like Astroglide, Gyne-Moistrin, Moist Again, Probe, and Aqualub, to name just a few on the market. Some brands like Wet or Eros market both a water-based or oil-based formula. Replens is a moisturizer and lubricant that helps restore a proper pH in the vagina as well as actually plumping up the tissue. Don't use oil-based petroleum jelly (Vaseline), as it doesn't clear easily from tissue and can result in infection. Women who are sensitive to yeast infections should also avoid the oil-based preparations.

Daily intake of zinc (15 mg), vitamin E (400 IUs), essential fatty acids (salmon, tuna, evening primrose oil, black currant seed oil), and other herbal extracts can often help improve lubrication.[4] When possible, avoid the substances that dry up membranes, such as antihistamines, diuretics, alcohol, and caffeine, as they also will dry the lining of the vagina. And don't forget to drink eight glasses of water a day.

Dyspareunia (Painful Intercourse)

This is the most common sexual complaint in older women. It's not hard to understand why this may be the case, with the loss of a cushioned vagina that is also less lubricated. Changes in the vaginal mucous membrane can increase one's vulnerability to infections that can provoke pain during intercourse. In addition, pain may be the result of a change in uterine contractions. The uterus experiences atrophy as a result of lower estrogen levels, so during orgasm, the uterine muscle contractions that used to be smooth and pleasurable become more spastic and painful.[5] Again, estrogen replacement will often restore full sexual functioning without pain for many of these problems. Estrogen replacement and other options when ERT is not possible or recommended will be discussed at more length in the next chapter.

Decrease in Frequency of Sexual Desire

As we mentioned earlier, there can be significant individual variation in how aging impacts desire and sexual frequency in women. What seems to account for the difference? Testosterone, in women as well as in men, seems to be "the libido hormone." It is likely that some of the desire changes in women are linked to a fall in testosterone, since the level of this hormone also drops along with estrogen. If a woman experiences low levels of sexual desire in the absence of relational problems or conflict, she should be encouraged to ask her physician to have her free testosterone level checked. If it is in the low range of normal, she may benefit from testosterone replacement. It can be formulated as a cream to be applied in the vulval area (but not before intercourse), or applied as a gel to the shoulders.

RELATIONAL ADJUSTMENTS

These physical symptoms of aging may diminish sexual enthusiasm and comfort in lovemaking. Couples will need to creatively address these issues for intercourse to be possible, let alone enjoyable. Because arousal and lubrication will often take longer, it is important for the couple to use the extra time to create an atmosphere that facilitates loveplay on this more relaxed journey into intimacy. Intercourse may need to be gentler at first and care taken on entry. Artificial lubrication ceases to be optional, as more liberal and frequent applications are necessary to counteract some of these physical changes. The husband may need to be more charming and alert to what pleasures his wife, so she feels cared for and open to his sexual advances.

It may take longer to reach orgasm, and its intensity and duration can diminish. However, even if the orgasm is less intense and takes more time to occur, a woman's ability to have multiple orgasms remains the same with age and, unlike in men, her refractory period does not extend.[6] With aging, he will need more time also, so this becomes a great time for the couple to relax and explore each other's bodies and begin to discover what each enjoys.

A difficult paradox exists with regard to female sexual changes and intercourse. On the one hand, regular sexual activity can contribute to a delay or reduction in the physical effects that begin at midlife. Sex enhances vaginal lubrication, reduces vaginal thinning, maintains the muscle tone of the vagina, and increases the blood supply to the vagina, helping to prevent atrophy. Women who have sexual intercourse once or twice a week before, during, and after menopause also tend to have fewer sexual dysfunctions.[7] The paradox is that it is often difficult "to use it or lose it" if one is experiencing painful intercourse, infections, vaginal dryness, low energy, sleep disturbances, depression, concern about attractiveness due to a change in body image, and over- all lowered sexual desire.

To resolve this paradox will require regular and clear communication with patience and understanding between partners. The majority of complaints concerning sexual- ity in aging adults are produced by a lack of knowledge of the normal physiological changes linked with age and an inability to communicate needs and preferences. Women, in particular, have difficulty identifying and expressing their sexual needs.[8]

When it comes to sexual response, perhaps even more significant than the physical and hormonal changes a woman experiences with aging is what occurs in her thoughts, feelings, and relationships. The combination of menopause, the changing roles of an empty nest, and an inability to have an orgasm can cause some wives to come to the erroneous conclusion that they are "too tired" or "too old" for sex. Many times this is because sex is perceived by the woman as another instance where someone is taking from her and she is not receiving a tangible benefit. Everyone tires of constantly giving when there is little received in return. This mind-set will pollute her perspective on sex, and her spouse will need to be very involved in restoring her joy.

Many women may struggle with long-standing sexual inhibitions, have experienced sexual abuse or victimiza- tion, have fears about losing their attractiveness, or be in an unsatisfactory relationship. Perhaps after many years of marriage, predictability has replaced spontaneity, and sex has become routine and mechanical. Sex therapy or counseling may be helpful in these situations.

So much of sex is in the head. This can be a rich time for you sexually; you have lost some of your earlier inhibitions and know more about what arouses you. Pregnancy is no longer a fear. You may have to engage in some self-talk about your attractiveness as your body loses its firmness and skin tone decreases. Again, maturity can be associated with greater skills and more comfortable attitudes. Older women make great lovers, but they may need their partners to help convince them of this fact.

Remember how we began this discussion: "I am woman, hear me roar." As you work to accept the many physical changes in your life, what kind of roar will be heard from you?

Chapter 4

Hope for Hormone Hostages?:
The Confusion of Menopausal Changes

*P*erhaps the question may be: Who is the "hostage" when hormones seem to be out of control? Wives certainly didn't choose this path. But quite often husbands comment, "I have been a hostage to my wife's hormones for years." Both partners are tremendously impacted. As a couple, we [Jim and Carolyn] became interested in this topic out of self-defense when Carolyn began experiencing some fairly significant peri-menopausal symptoms. It became imperative to understand more about what was happening to her physiologically, and also the impact emotionally, psychologically, sexually, and spiritually.

We have discovered it to be not only an experiential process, but an *experimental* one as well. As we talk with couples who are dealing with hormonal changes and fluctuations, we find that this journey may begin with PMS in the teenage years, move into perimenopausal symptoms as early as age thirty-five, move on through menopause at an average age of fifty-two, and finally reach postmenopause. Hormonal fluctuations occur throughout most of a woman's life, requiring her (and her spouse) to make many adjustments and accommodations both personally and relationally.

Menopause is the time in life that the female ceases to have a menstrual cycle and the possibility of pregnancy is over. It is defined as having occurred when a woman goes twelve months without a period. Basically, estrogen dwindles so low that it can no longer "tell" the body to menstruate. If one wanted to assess with blood tests whether they were experiencing menopause, you would look for a pattern of increasing follicle stimulating hormone (FSH) and decreasing estradiol. Menopause "naturally" occurs between the ages of forty-five and fifty-five (average 51.4 years), yet it can begin as early as in the thirties or as late as the sixties, and can be "induced" if a woman has had a hysterectomy (removal of the uterus and possibly the ovaries). Cigarette smokers and former smokers can reach menopause two years earlier than nonsmokers.

Perimenopause is the transition between fertility and the last menstrual period. It can begin as early as age thirty-five but generally begins in the midforties. There may be some overlap in symptoms with regard to perimenopause and menopause, as one may notice irregular menstrual patterns, hot flashes and night sweats, corresponding to changes in estrogen levels. Other common symptoms include vaginal inelasticity and/or dryness, urinary incontinence, insomnia, fatigue, loss of concentration and memory lapses, skin changes, gray hair (or hair loss, including that in the pubic area), and formication (a perception of skin crawling, a prickly feeling, or a feeling of bugs biting you).[1]

Although it has not been shown to be directly related to menopause, periodic depression and an increase in headaches are common, as well as dizziness, heart palpitations, and anxiety. If a person is predisposed to headaches, the headaches can be worse during this time, as migraines can be triggered by hormonal changes. Weight gain is also common because of slower basal metabolism. The degree to which women experience symptoms depends on how much and how fast their estrogen levels drop, their testosterone levels, their genetic predisposition to aging (i.e., how did your mother age?), one's overall health, their continued sexual activity and enjoyment, the diligence with which they exercise their vaginal muscles, and their attitudes about aging, sex, and this stage of life.[2]

Many of these symptoms can affect a wife's motivation for sex and her self-esteem, which are intertwined. With all of the physical changes, women need a positive attitude and crucial spousal support to cope with menopause. Some points of encouragement: Research suggests that women consistently feel relief when menstruation ends, and postmenopausal women have a more positive view of menopause than do perimenopausal women. Wives do not feel they become less sexually attractive after menopause. For some the freedom can enhance sexual desire and increase frequency of love-making. It is important that women not associate repro-ductive ability with sexual ability. (These are two separate functions, and you can have one without the other.)

HORMONES AND SEXUALITY

Estrogen, progesterone, and testosterone are the chief hormones involved in cycles of female sexuality. Considerable controversy surrounds the use of hormone replacement therapies (testosterone for men and increas-ingly for women, and estrogen or a combination of estrogen/progesterone for women). This chapter will discuss primarily the effects these hormones have on sexuality and will present the options without endorsing a particular approach. That decision should be made in consultation with your medical doctor and with consid-eration to recent research. Research in this area is chang-ing quickly and information gained two to three years ago may now be out of date.

Estrogen

Levels of estrogen and sexual desire do not seem to be correlated, and sex drive fluctuations across the men-strual cycle do not seem to be related to estrogen levels.[3] In fact, many women find their sexual desire increases when estrogen levels drop, because the ratio of *testosterone* (the strongest hormone of sexual desire in a group of chemicals called androgens) to female hormones is proportionally greater.

Estrogen replacement therapy (ERT) can provide relief from some of the psychological and physical problems associated with menopause, and thus indirectly enhance sexual response. Possible improvements include a renewed sense of well-being, a decrease in anxiety, fewer sleep disruptions (because of reduced hot flashes and cold sweats), improved genital sensation, an increase in blood flow and thickening of the vaginal wall, and improved vaginal lubrication. Estrogens promote dream sleep, during which time secretions may "irrigate" the vagina.

Women who do not suffer from painful intercourse (due to vaginal atrophy and problems with lubrication) will benefit little from estrogen replacement.[4] However, if a woman is suffering from decreased sexual desire, natural, plant-based estrogen creams now formulated by many companies are available in health food stores. Another option may be a transdermal estrogen formula (a skin patch). The good news with "the patch" is that unlike pills, it doesn't appear to raise blood levels of a protein linked to increased risk for heart disease.[5] The full benefits of ERT in relation to improved sexual desire, however, are reliably achieved only with the addition of testosterone.

Progesterone

Provera and other brands of progesterone are utilized in replacement therapy along with estrogen in order to regulate the menstrual cycle. It may help to prevent uterine cancer by allowing cells in the uterine lining to slough off periodically in the form of a period. An increase in the level of progesterone throughout the menstrual cycle has been associated with decreased sexual desire, primarily due to its tendency to reduce testosterone levels. Progesterone also has the tendency to cause depression, inhibit orgasm, and may lower DHEA (another plentiful androgen, but less potent than testosterone in sexual desire; androgens create desire and have steroid effects in muscle and hair growth). Progesterone is associated with reduced physical sensitivity, and it functions as a sedative in moderate doses and as an anesthetic at high doses.[6]

However, there are some women who may benefit from the use of a transdermal 2 percent progesterone cream, because natural progesterone can turn into androgens and even a form of estrogen when the body needs more of these hormones. It is important to note that the body functions best when there is an appropriate balance among the sex hormones. Often, sexual difficulties or emotional instability are the result of too much or too little of one or more of these hormones.

What About the Women's Health Initiative Study?

In the last year, many older women who had been on hormone replacement therapy were taken off supplemental hormones by their doctors, based on research findings in the Women's Health Initiative Study. Many of these women had functioned quite well on hormones for years and began to experience the effects of withdrawal from estrogen. Exactly how great was the increased risk for heart disease, breast cancer, stroke, and blood clots in the study? The researchers found that, out of

10,000 women, an additional 7 would have heart attacks, 8 more would have breast cancer, 8 more would have a stroke, and 18 more would have blood clots. That may be considered a fairly small increased risk. However, women should discuss this added risk, along with their family medical history, personal medical history, and any other risk factors, with their doctors. The researchers looked at the effects of Prempro, a high-dose combination of estrogen and progestin. Studies are continuing for women who are on estrogen alone.[7]

Side effects of taking estrogen include nausea, headaches, and bloating. Progesterone can produce the PMS-like symptoms of fluid retention, moodiness, breast tenderness, and headaches. HRT can cause hypertension, liver and blood-clotting problems, and increase the risk of breast cancer. You are a poor candidate for HRT if you have or had: a previous diagnosis of breast or endometrial cancer; blood clots, phlebitis, or uterine fibroids; gallbladder disease or liver disease.

A recent study has revealed that about a quarter of women who stop taking HRT because of its risks wind up resuming the pills because of menopause misery.[8] Women who really need estrogen, especially if they're otherwise at low risk of heart disease or cancer, shouldn't be scared away from it. Female doctors don't seem to be. A new poll of American College of Obstetricians and Gynecologists members found half of female OB/GYNs who are bothered by menopause use some form of hormone therapy themselves. The key is taking as little as possible for as short a period as possible.

Desperate for alternatives to alleviate hot flashes, more

women are turning to certain antidepressants, such as those in the Prozac family and Effexor, which can offer some relief even if the user isn't depressed. This option isn't widely known but is slowly gaining interest. In that OB/GYN poll, 13 percent of menopause-bothered doctors said they are trying antidepressants. Nobody knows why they work. But small studies suggest the antidepressants reduce hot flashes by about 60 percent, not as good as estrogen although better than other options so far have proved. Doses are half or even less of the starting dose for depression treatment, so low that side effects mostly are decreased libido and some weight fluctuation.

Selective estrogen receptor modulators (SERMs) like raloxifene may provide another alternative to conventional HRT in women with increased risk for breast or uterine cancer or for those unable to tolerate conventional HRT. In addition, other natural remedies should be pursued. *The Menopause Manager* by Mary Ann and Joseph Mayo is an excellent resource for further ideas in this area.[9]

Testosterone

In the female, the ovaries produce some testosterone, with additional testosterone being derived from the adrenal steroids. Removal of the ovaries will decrease sexual desire to a certain extent. Testosterone treatment seems to be useful in facilitating sexual desire in a subset of women with low sexual desire, but it requires safety monitoring, and there are not clearly defined dosage levels for females.[10] Several pharmacies now prepare a 1 percent to 2 percent testosterone cream that can be applied to the vulval area once or twice daily (but not prior to intercourse). Studies have shown that women with higher testosterone levels reported less depression, experienced more sexual gratification with their husbands, and showed a greater capacity to form good interpersonal relationships. Testosterone also seems to increase clitoral sensitivity.[11]

In addition to seeing your gynecologist, you may need to consult an endocrinologist who specializes in hormonal treatment to discuss whether you may benefit from some form of hormone replacement. All women who are seeking treatment for diminished sex drive should have their testosterone and DHEA levels measured. In those women who don't seem to be able to produce enough of their own androgens, DHEA or testosterone can be given in the form of a skin cream, a gel, or a capsule. If both levels are low, it may be a good idea to try replenishing DHEA first (10–25 mg a day). It is a precursor to testosterone and can increase testosterone levels by one and a half to two times. The dosing for testosterone replacement for those who don't respond to DHEA is not clearly defined and will depend on the woman's individual needs and/or blood levels. The side effects of testosterone replacement in women are usually extra hair growth, skin changes, and, in rare cases, a lowering of the voice. Testosterone can also decrease HDL (good) cholesterol levels.

Collect as much information as possible and be an advocate for your own health care. There is no magical answer, pill, prayer, exercise, or diet. And, in all likelihood, the more you research this topic, the more confused you will become. As you read and study hormone replacement options, it may seem the question often is: "Well, it looks like you can take your choice, either uterine cancer or breast cancer. Which do you want?" Or you will meet people who say, "This is what really worked for me," or "I found this natural remedy. It does this, this, and this." The difficulty is that a remedy or intervention *may not work the same for each person*. The whole body is complex ("fearfully and wonderfully made"), and it is also unique. What works well for one person may only be effective for a short period of time or may actually increase symptoms for someone else. Keep in mind that each treatment has to be *tailored* to that person, and collecting as much information as possible is imperative, especially about the medication or herbals that are being taken. When one's hormones are fluctuating widely, the chances increase that even the rare side effects of a medication may impact you. If you choose to pursue hormone replacement, it helps to have someone come alongside (a physician, a therapist, or spouse) who can help you begin to sort through the symptoms and the options.

The combination of genetics, general health, and personal life experience makes each woman's menopause unique. For the woman who experiences very little impact from the "change of life," blessings on you. But for the many women (and their spouses) who find menopause to be a confusing time replete with irregular periods, hot flashes, erratic moods, sleeplessness, fatigue, depression, and pain, sexual challenges will result.

Husbands are an essential component in the coping

process. They can certainly help to make things better or they can clearly make matters worse. We have talked to a number of women about what they need or what they wish their spouses would do for them when they are experiencing some specific perimenopausal or menopausal problems. We have received a myriad of responses, such as, "Direct the children in their responsibilities so I don't have to think all the time," "Sympathize, listen, and be concerned instead of always trying to 'fix' me," "Stop and hug me during a temper tantrum. Don't run away or choose to be disagreeable." Men often miss that when a woman seems to be the most unlovable is when she most needs to be loved. When a woman is emotionally all over the board it may feel as if you are trying to hug a porcupine—yet that is often what she needs the most.

A third of a woman's life will be postmenopausal. But remember, "This, too, shall pass!" Hope for the future exists as we embrace this challenge and apply creative solutions.

Time Out: Husbands, work with your wife in making a list of the top three problems she is encountering and be a part of the creative solutions for each.

Chapter 5

Performance Power or Passionate Partner?:
Male Sexual Changes

*M*en, how much of your sexual self-esteem is contained between your legs? If your answer is "Not that much," then let me ask another question: "Have you named your penis?" Rarely does a day go by that I [Jim] don't receive spam e-mail touting penis patches, pills, and potions. The advertising would be laughable if this media blitz didn't result in apparent sales. The ads promise "massive" growth in length, girth, and stamina for your "tool." The messages promote the notion that "bigger is better," that the penis has an identity of its own, and to have less than a rock-solid erection is embarrassingly unmanly.

What is the message to those of us who are aging? Unless we hold on to youthful firmness in our erections and actually increase their length, we are sexual failures. This media barrage and type of advertising is incredulous to me in its immaturity, and it demeans masculinity. I don't believe a pill promoting "penis performance power" will reverse the aging process or make me a "passionate partner." Dr. Barry Bass referred to this phenomenon as the "sexual performance perfection industry (SPPI)," and he describes this concept as follows:

> The message of the SPPI is designed to create feelings of inadequacy and to remind men (and women) that we do not "measure up" and that we never will unless we become regular consumers of the industry's products . . . [The implication is that] good sex equals intercourse and requires a hard penis that stays erect throughout a sexual encounter. This definition of "good sex" changes the basic nature of a sexual encounter from one of intimacy and pleasure to one of achievement and performance.[1]

Both men and women struggle with the aging process and the effects it has on their sexuality. Though it shouldn't be true, our culture discriminates against the aging person. A man's ego is affected by performance. Concepts like strength, stamina, production, and physical prowess are valued. Many centuries ago the philosopher Descartes avowed, "I think, therefore I am." Many men continue to believe that one's very existence and value, both personal and sexual, is more accurately viewed as "I am erect, therefore I am." This man will naturally be concerned as he experiences aging and normal changes in sexual performance. He may wonder about his erection not being as firm and requiring more stimulation to achieve it. In youth he could look at a nude body and instantly get firm. Occasionally, now he experiences some degree of impotence (or what is now referred to as erectile dysfunction), failure to achieve an ejaculation, or prevention of some activities due to an aching back and muscles. He begins to question if he will continue to enjoy sexual pleasure and be able to bring true enjoyment to his partner.

PHYSICAL CHANGES

As you get older, there is normal wear and tear on your body's nerves, muscles, and blood supply, which can affect sexual functioning. You may have to ease off on certain positions. Quality and quantity of your erections and orgasms may change. That does not make you impotent or sexually inadequate. With a better understanding of yourself, you'll have the freedom for greater enjoyment with less anxiety. Be reassured that lovemaking will continue to be good. Here are five common changes a man experiences with the aging process:

1. *Erections will require more direct physical stimulation of the penis.* In younger years, visual or mental sexual stimuli could bring about an erection. That doesn't mean you are losing your sexual desire because your wife's breasts or genitals don't create the same quick reflex action. Sometimes this can mistakenly be seen as dysfunction because both partners expect spontaneous reactions as in the past. When enjoying love play and wanting to engage in intercourse, you and your partner

will have to touch and play with the penis. If you lose some or all of your erection, while focusing on pleasuring your wife, more direct stimulation will be required to get the penis firm again.

Like other aspects of aging, this does not have to be a serious problem. Husbands, these changes are normal, so don't blame or be angry with your mate. You and your wife must not interpret the lack of instant arousal as any reflection on her attractiveness. It is physiological, and she can simply make a note to engage in more manual and oral stimulation of the penis. Sometimes it can be arousing to stuff the partially erect penis into the vagina manually, as enough erection is gained to enjoy intercourse. Both of you can be erotically aroused as you make adjustments and, in a loving, sensual way, creatively stimulate the male organ.

2. *The penis may not achieve the same firmness with erections.* With aging, the blood supply can be diminished, and the muscle valve system that keeps the blood in the penis can have leakage. The penis therefore will not achieve the same hardness as before. I have spoken to many middle-aged men who were very concerned that they were experiencing erectile dysfunction because the angle of the erect penis had changed. "It used to be at two o'clock and now it's barely four thirty." This change can evolve into more of an attitude problem than a real issue. The penis does not need to be extra firm; it simply needs to be hard enough to insert and thrust. This condition is made worse if one is a smoker, because nicotine promotes arterial damage in the penis as well as other parts of the body, and the valve system that holds blood

in the penis is even more compromised. In a sense, then, smoking will prematurely age the penis.[2]

I'm reminded of a story: An elderly man went for his annual physical exam and related to his physician, "Doc, when I was twenty my erections were rock solid. When I got into my forties I could begin to bend them half an inch, in my sixties I could push it an inch, and now in my eighties I can flex it almost two inches. Isn't it amazing how much stronger I am at eighty-three?"

Like this gentleman, don't let your attitude get in the way. The firmness of erections does not make the man; it is not the symbol of a great lover. The surest way to become psychologically impotent is to worry about erections rather than enjoy the moment. During some lovemaking sessions you may not achieve an erection, or you may achieve only partial firmness. Don't worry about it. Chalk it up to fatigue and distractions, and know the erection will come back. (You may want to read the section in Chapter 8 that deals with erectile difficulties.) Your wife can be helpful in reducing your anxiety. Sometimes you may enjoy a penis that is not firm enough for intercourse, but can be pleasured through to an orgasm. You can mentally destroy your lovemaking by worrying about your firmness.

This point affects only a man who has not been circumcised. With aging, the skin of the foreskin may lose some of its elasticity and tighten. Full erections and intercourse may cause the skin to split, rather than stretch as it once did. These skin tears will be small and will heal quickly, but they can be painful. Pulling back the foreskin at night before going to sleep can often prevent this condition. During the sleep cycle and nightly erections, the skin will be stretched and be less likely to split during subsequent erections.

The bottom line is that a little shrinkage over time is normal. If this is any consolation, in some men the scrotal sac stretches and hangs lower, which can make sitting on the toilet a refreshing experience. Another complicating factor is that as we age and add more weight in the waist area, the penis can become absorbed more into fat tissue and become more difficult to view over the stomach. Refuse to let your ego and value as a man be tied into your penis, or you will have a problem as you get older. If you must continue to observe and fret about your penis size, might I suggest using your wife's makeup mirror. The extra magnification may offer you an improved perspective and soothe your battered self-image. Then again, diet and exercise may not hurt either.

3. *The waiting time between erections/ejaculations will increase, with climaxes needed less often.* Men are different from women and need what is called a refractory time to rest between orgasms. Some women are multiorgasmic even into older age and can be stimulated to a climax several times in a row. When you were nineteen, your refractory period was less than a minute, but it may be a day or more as you get into your sixties. Both partners need to consider this. Don't panic or create feelings of anxiety or failure by attempting to create another erection and orgasm before the body has had enough recuperative time.

Remember that making love does not depend on an erection or an orgasm. Enjoy each other, and if an erection or orgasm is difficult to achieve, your body may be recovering. Be creative and enjoy intimacy as you help your partner achieve her climax. If you have not climaxed and you are focusing on your partner and lose your erection, this is not a refractory period. Apply direct stimulation and you will most likely regain your erection.

As you age into your sixties and seventies, you may need to climax only once a week or once or twice a month. That does not mean sexual closeness with your wife two or three times a week will be impossible, but remember, lovemaking is a mutual endeavor and may also involve cuddling, caressing, and holding, and not always intercourse. You should not push yourself to climax every time there is intercourse. Putting pressure on yourself to perform and achieve certain results can result in anxiety and loss of erections.

4. Ejaculation is less strong, and erections disappear more quickly. With aging, you may not feel quite as much like a volcano going off at your climax. The muscles that expel the semen are less strong, but that does not have to affect the pleasure of an orgasm. Part of the explosion-like feeling is in your head and has nothing to do with the expulsion of semen. Again, I have spoken with men that "used to be able to hit the ceiling" with their ejaculations and now are concerned with what seems like a "dribble." Relax, ejaculations are not meant for target practice, but for pleasure and release. Building greater sexual tension during lovemaking, accumulating more semen, and letting yourself mentally focus on your orgasm as you build toward the edge and then abandon yourself to the feelings, create stronger orgasms.

After you climax, you may find yourself losing the erection faster than in years past. Don't let that affect the afterglow as you hold each other and share closeness. If your penis doesn't stay in your wife's vagina, caress and hug and hold her as you tell her how much pleasure she brings you sexually. Learn not to worry about seepage of semen from the vagina, but sensually and emotionally enjoy each other in intimate ways.

5. *The pleasure of intercourse can be longer.* This is a pleasant outcome of needing less ejaculation and fewer climaxes. Don't put pressure on yourself to have an orgasm; some lovemaking sessions may be enjoyed with other types of pleasuring. With your added endurance, you can last longer and the active thrusting can pleasure your wife. It is important to be sensitive to her pleasure needs, which may not always require longer, active thrusting. Your wife's vagina has less padding as she gets older, so prolonged thrusting can become painful.

You may want to use certain positions (e.g., wife-on-top) that let your wife be more active. This is a great time to experiment and play at this aspect of making love. There are advantages to growing older.

HORMONAL CHANGES
AND SEXUALITY

Testosterone is the primary sex hormone influencing sexual desire in both males and females. Women need a small amount for sexual desire, compared to men who have higher levels of testosterone produced by the testicles in addition to the adrenal gland. However, this does not mean men will always have a higher sexual desire. In men, the primary effect of lower testosterone is reduced sex drive rather than the inability to get an erection. In fact, testosterone replacement is clinically effective for sex drive only in men who are low in testosterone. It is not prescribed for men complaining of erection problems and normal libido.

Is There Really a Male Menopause?

There has been much discussion in the last few years debating the evidence for a "male menopause" to describe the physical, psychological, and emotional changes many men experience after midlife. Just as we discussed in the previous chapter regarding the female menopause, the aging and hormonal change process is not the same for all men, although it is also not nearly as abrupt or significant for men as it is for women. What is commonly referred to as male menopause is probably the net effect of at least three "pauses"—andropause, adrenopause, and somatopause.

The process of the gradual decline in levels of testosterone in men is called *andropause*. This testosterone decline doesn't have the same impact and is not as rapid as the estrogen loss that women experience. In men ages forty to eighty, the decrease in total serum testosterone is about 0.4 percent a year. The decline begins to increase after age sixty, but there is considerable individual variability and andropause is not noticeable in all men. Some men will remain sexually active into their eighties and nineties, although the frequency may be somewhat lower than when they were in their forties and fifties. The symptoms associated with andropause can include a lack of energy, fatigue or listlessness; diminished productivity and a disinclination to work; decreases in muscle, bone mass, libido, and appetite; poor concentration and memory; physical hypersensitivity; and increased irritability and sometimes depression.[3]

If there is severely limited desire or persistent impotence or inability to ejaculate, have your physician check your blood and hormone levels, including serum testosterone, complete blood count (CBC), prostate specific antigen (PSA), and basic serum chemistries. If a low testosterone level is discovered, you may be a candidate for testosterone replacement, which can be in pill form, injections, implants, patches, or gels. The gel form, which absorbs through the skin, has become a popular means of treatment due to its ease in application and in the ability to adjust doses. You should begin to see some improvement in sexual functioning within a two-week period. However, desire may begin to increase sooner, and is generally necessary for achieving an erection. Remember that increasing libido does not necessarily result in improved sexual performance or an improved relationship. Testosterone is just part of the story; it is not a panacea for all sexual or relational ills.

It is important to be under the care of a physician because there can be certain side effects like water retention, an aggravation of high blood pressure, and an enlarging of the prostate. If the testosterone level is too high, anger and aggressive behavior will increase. Certain conditions, such as prostate cancer, would contraindicate the use of testosterone replacement therapy. Keep your doctor informed regarding any effects of treatment, be they positive or negative.

A second "pause" occurs as the adrenocortical cells responsible for the production of the steroid dehydro-epiandrosterone (DHEA) decrease in activity; this is experienced as *adrenopause*. At age thirty, DHEA levels are five times higher than at age eighty-five. DHEA appears to be a "healthy" steroid that enhances quality of life and may promote longevity. It appears to only be associated with sex drive in women but functions in both sexes to protect the immune system, inhibit tumors, and promote bone growth. A decline in DHEA levels could thus be a catalyst for illness and aging. Research studies seem to support the value of DHEA supplementation (50–100 mg daily) in increasing perceived psychological and physical well-being and in improving lean body mass and body strength in men. Since it is an androgen (although with only about 3 percent the potency of testosterone), the scientific verdict is still out as to the negative long-term effects that DHEA supplementation may have on prostate or other forms of cancer.[4]

The final "pause" involves the decrease in growth hormone (GH) released by the pituitary gland in the brain, which causes a decrease in the production of an insulin-like growth factor (IGF-I) in the liver. The result is referred to as *somatopause*, which seems to be associated with a decline in one's functional capacity (decrease in muscle mass and strength, bone strength, and quality of life).[5] This appears to be a very normal consequence of aging, yet many men are gulping supplements that contain various forms of human growth hormone. Research has not yet validated the long-term positive effect of this strategy, let alone the potential negative effects.

Aging is as inevitable as death and taxes. The process will bring about male sexual changes. We can fight getting older and pursue the perfectly powerful penis, or we can accept and value our physical changes. Let's seek to make the kinds of adjustments that will allow us to be genuine lovers and passionate partners.

Chapter 6

"You Are So Beautiful to Me":
Redeeming Body Image

ere I am. It's 5:30 A.M. and I can't sleep. I [Carolyn] heave my sleep-deprived body into the bathroom. Yikes! The mirror reflects a female with bags under her eyes and a less-than-perfect coiffure. (Hot flashes—or power surges—in the night are not conducive to lovely morning hair!) A closer look reveals at least two extra wrinkles, and the low-fat yogurt I consumed last night seems to have been lathered on my hips, somehow managing to avoid the digestive process altogether. My leg is aching, and as I look down, I note a varicose vein has materialized overnight. It definitely looks colorful amid the spider veins and the cellulite dimples. What is the deal? I eat healthy, even include lots of soy. I swim five or six times a week. My cupboard is filled with supplements that I take regularly. Who is this woman? And how did the athletic, slender woman of twenty or thirty or even forty years turn into this?

In the midst of my musings, my husband comes in. At this point I begin to show him all my discoveries. He sympathizes with me, but then adds, "You sure look beautiful to me!" Has he lost his eyesight? Or have I lost my mind?

Many of us recall Joe Cocker's rendition of "You Are So Beautiful." Even though some may think he sounds like a croaking bullfrog, the message of the song is simple and touching. "You are so beautiful to me, *can't you see* . . . You're everything I hope for, you're everything I need . . . You are so beautiful to me." The problem for many women is that they "can't see."

BODY IMAGE AND ATTITUDES

Body image is all about what happens in the mind, not in the mirror. Remember, our most powerful sex organ is our brain. That's where it all begins. When we see ourselves as unattractive, we assume our partner sees us that way as well. After all, we wouldn't want to go to bed with ourselves, and as a result, we've just dampened our desire and interest in anything sexual.

We generally form our attitudes about our body from the people and ideas around us. Look at the following list. How have these influences affected the way you think and feel? Think about different parts of your body—your hair, mouth, legs, stomach, chest, genitals— and sort through how each influence has affected the way you perceive yourself.

- Media—television, movies, videos, songs, books, newspapers, and magazines
- Family—family values, comments, body shapes, interactions with siblings, parents, and grandparents
- Peers—friends, schoolmates, work associates, opposite-sex and same-sex influences
- Church and religious beliefs—sermons, comments, type of dress and conduct, and biblical interpretations
- Significant adults—Scout leader or youth minister, teacher, neighbor, boss, or friend of family
- Dates or romantic interests—group dating, individual dates, boyfriends/girlfriends, or previous spouse

Which of the above affected you most in your attitudes about your body as a young person, and which of them are still impacting you in midlife or beyond?

Now think for a moment about the people you have known who were or are older than fifty. How have they affected how you perceive this time of your life? Most people have a skewed perception of aging. It may be faulty in many ways. In this era, we are constantly subjected to the picture the media have painted for us—one of prizing youth, slimness, and being forever young. In addition, many baby boomers and their offspring believe that the rules (including aging) do not really apply to them. Boomers are very comfortable thinking outside the box and achieving new goals. Is all of this unrealistic? Not necessarily, provided we face the truth that aging can't be avoided. A realistic approach must include knowing and understanding aging.

The apostle Paul sums up the mind-set that we must adopt in 2 Corinthians 4:16: "Our physical body is becoming older and weaker, but our spirit inside us is made new every day" (NCV). Aging is inevitable, but we have a choice as to our response to the process. In fact, the response we choose will greatly impact our self-perception and our relationships with our partners, our longevity, and our sexual functioning.

BODY IMAGE AND EXPECTATIONS

The cosmetic surgeons are kept busy making breasts bigger or smaller, tightening vaginas, removing wrinkles, eliminating sags, and liposuctioning fat. How we feel about ourselves definitely affects our ability to relax and enjoy making love with abandon and pleasure. *Great lovers have grown to be comfortable and confident with their bodies and sexuality.*

In a major study, two-thirds of the women said they were affected sexually by one or more aspects of their body image. "Most women suffer from unrealistic expectations about how their bodies must look and must continue to look."[1] In a mystery novel I read recently, the villain is never suspected until the very end. At that point, one of the characters says the reason the person was not caught by their actions or their comments was "because no one notices older women. Unless you're beautiful like Laura, or pushy like me, or really famous in your field, no one sees you or listens to you . . . When we're old and plain, we become invisible."[2]

Unfortunately, there is much truth to this. Our culture

60

bombards women with so many unrealistic expectations and stereotypes of what is attractive and sensual, it
is no wonder more women than men get caught up in
these stereotypes. However, men can experience these
feelings too.

BODY IMAGE AND MATURITY

If this irrational notion represents "reality" in our culture, what can be done to correct it? Perhaps the following illustration will help.

I remember vividly my first visit to Willow Creek
Community Church in the northwestern suburbs of
Chicago. What a fabulous church facility—the latest
technology, well laid out and practical location of various
departments, easy access—it's difficult to imagine that
there could be any way to improve the place. I have also
visited other churches where a single room can function
as a gymnasium, worship center, multiple classrooms, or
a dining room. The efficiency and functionality of these
facilities are truly amazing.

I also recall on trips to Europe visiting some of the
most marvelous cathedrals in the world. You could
almost visualize the saints of long ago worshiping there.
In this case, it was often not easy to access; the facilities
(bathrooms in particular) were hard to locate and sometimes nonexistent. Some of the floors had been marred
by swords or horses hooves and blood from war—but
the gouges were no longer rough. They blended in to
form the character and aesthetic beauty, which was
enhanced by the light patterns woven in through the

stained-glass windows. The beauty was awesome. I never heard any of the visitors comment, "We should replace this gouged floor with a new scuff-resistant material." No, the beauty was enhanced because of the age. The "flaws" or "scars" were a testimony to the history of the place and memorialized events and people.

Which type of building is the best? It is obvious that they cannot be compared. Each has its own purpose; each has its own beauty; and each has its own place in time. Which facility is worth more? Again, there is not a standard to compare them. This, I believe, is a picture of what is happening to many people with regard to body image. The Sistine Chapel is not Willow Creek, and a fifty- or sixty-year-old body is not, nor will it ever be again, eighteen years old.

In many cultures, a special place of respect is given to aging individuals. Scripture also values aging as special: "Show respect to old people; stand up in their presence" (Lev. 19:32 NCV). Again in the New Testament we find that older women are to instruct the younger, attributing value and wisdom to aging (Titus 2:3-4).

BODY IMAGE AND ACCEPTANCE IN WOMEN AND MEN

This stage of life means being comfortable with who you are. Jennifer Lopez, one of Hollywood's "hot" women today, was recently interviewed by *Reader's Digest*. When asked what makes a woman sexy, she replied that it wasn't the breast size, curvy body, or lack of cellulite, but rather a certain air that shows the woman is comfortable with herself. She also stated that she hopes she has helped Hollywood change its definition of *beautiful.* "It's important for all types of women to know that you don't have to fit a prototype of what one person thinks is beautiful in order to be or feel beautiful."[3] Perhaps Ms. Lopez is actually restating a biblical principle: "No, your beauty should come from within you—the beauty of a gentle and quiet spirit that will never be destroyed" (1 Peter 3:4 NCV).

Much of this chapter has focused on encouraging women to age gracefully and see beauty in the process, because women tend to struggle with this more than men. Interestingly, older men are sometimes described as "distinguished" or "wise" as they begin to show signs of aging. The following cartoons show in an exaggerated way how men and women often see themselves compared to reality.

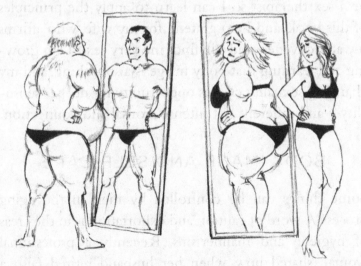

I [Doug] would not disagree with the fact that aging has been easier on me, and the above cartoon accurately portrays the ease with which men can take body image in stride. As I head toward sixty, I have to confess this has not been an easy decade. My sagging skin, the deterioration of muscle tone of my chest (not fun as it morphs into breasts), and growing stomach have made me sadly realize that I am more comfortable wearing a T-shirt at the beach. My intake of ibuprofen after exercise and the sore muscles the day after are an additional frustration. I guess I hoped I might avoid the normal physical effects of aging on my sexuality and body performance—but alas, I am very normal.

Somewhere deep in my masculine soul, with its need to perform competently and keep a competitive edge, I run scared. I don't always like what I see in the mirror, and the difference in ejaculating force or penis performance creates insecurity and challenges. I am grateful to be a sex therapist so I can learn to apply the principles of this book, and I am grateful for my wife, who affirms my attractiveness and still finds me very sexy. I am growing and learning that body image is a soul thing, and my changing sexuality creates opportunity for deeper sensuality—and different but intense arousal and connection.

BODY IMAGE AND SELF-CARE

Some things can be controlled by men in the aging process. A word of caution and exhortation is in the areas of hygiene and mannerisms. Recently a professional woman shared how when her husband retired (also a professional), he developed several annoying mannerisms—such as belching loudly and passing gas freely—

which she found embarrassing and really "turned her off." Another woman shared how her partner (in his seventies) was fastidious in his personal hygiene and grooming—even on the very day he passed away from kidney failure. His self-care made him attractive to her (twenty-five years his junior), even to the very end.

The sparkle and pizzazz will stay far longer in a marriage when both the man and woman practice good hygiene and general respect for their bodies. Too often we as humans forget to treat our bodies as "God's temple" (see 1 Cor. 3:16), whether it is a new "high-tech" model or an elegant timeless cathedral. When that is the care we give ourselves and the vision we have of ourselves, we will be more prepared to engage in intimacy with our partner. We will be able to state as the husband said to his wife in the mystery novel referred to earlier, "As long as I'm alive you will never be invisible—or plain—or old. Love has very clear eyes about things like that."

BODY IMAGE AND AFFIRMATION

In concluding this chapter, let us make some practical suggestions for both men and women as to how we can maturely look through the eyes of love and enhance our own and our partner's body image.

1. Body image at any age, but especially after fifty, comes down to our mental perceptions, our cognitive attitudes. "Our physical body is becoming older and weaker, but our spirit inside us is made new every day" (2 Cor. 4:16 NCV). "Do not change yourselves to be like the people of this world, but be changed within by a new way of thinking" (Rom.

12:2 NCV). The aging process is inevitable, but we have a choice as to our response. We can dispute our false beliefs and affirm the truth. Create some affirmations and let them resonate in your thinking: "Maturity is sensual and experienced." "We carry in our bodies the mementos of life."

2. Value and affirm your partner's masculinity or femininity on a deeper soul level. This can have a wonderful impact on body image. I [Doug] may not wrestle all the heavy bags around at the airport anymore, but I take charge of the porters doing that and flag down the taxi. My wife will make statements like, "You're so smart and strong; I like the way you take care of me." Affirmations motivate us to take the initiative.

3. Put your best foot forward. After a mastectomy, women are told to strategically utilize a camisole to lessen visual impact. As we age, we can strategically use lighting, clothing, and props to promote sensuality and minimize self-consciousness. Being partially clothed may engage our imagination more than total nudity. Some positions of intercourse, or lying flat on the bed may be more comfortable and flattering. Don't feel bad; models also avoid certain positions in being photographed. Let playfulness abound, and erotically look through the eyes of love.

What a wonderful vocation and responsibility mates have in affirming their partner's body image. We make a profound difference in how sensual they feel and their openness to lovemaking. Wives, believe your husbands. "You are so beautiful to me, *can't you see* . . . You're everything I hope for, you're everything I need . . . You are so beautiful to me."

Chapter 7

Lost in the Labyrinth of Life:
Coping with Changing Roles

*I*t's Friday night and you're looking forward to some time together at the close of a busy week. The phone rings and your mother informs you that your father has just been diagnosed with cancer. Your college-age son has been in a serious car accident five states away (car's totaled; he's fine). One daughter is crying on the phone because she and her boyfriend are fighting. The other daughter calls with a change of plans due to a rescheduled school event. Your twelve-year-old twin sons are arguing because one wants to attend a church social and the other wants to have a "sleepover." The cat is sick and needs medication every two hours. Today the doctor drained a cyst in your breast, which is now bruised and a brilliant shade of purple and blue. Tonight your husband begins his "prep" for a colonoscopy. Feeling sexy yet? (I bet that's what Job and his wife thought too.) Welcome to the "labyrinth of life"!

Someone once said that "the only stress-free environment is death." Midlife and beyond introduces us to a multitude of changes, and change involves stress. Stress on our bodies and stress on our relationships. It is a popular concept to refer to "midlife crises," but this phenomenon actually occurs throughout life. They might be better titled "identity" or "purpose in life" struggles. They all involve realizing goals and dreams, facing mortality, and creating deeper intimacy. Areas usually included are sexuality, relationships, spirituality, career and life pursuits, and meaningful leisure distractions.

Sex after fifty has to consider not only the physical changes but also the midlife relational changes that occur in the crucial years leading up to and including retirement. Middle age keeps getting pushed back, so I am not sure what middle age is anymore. For this chapter, a definition of midlife is not crucial because we are examining the sexual cycles of a couple's life from the midforties to eighty (or older) where much reevaluating goes on. During these years, we constantly reassess many parts of ourselves that have great impact on our sex lives: intimate companionship, sexual passion and variety, career development and retirement, and children in later stages of leaving the nest (notice I said stages of leaving the nest because I don't think they ever do completely).

Sex is different as we age and our marriages mature. That does not mean we give sex less priority or lose our intimate passion. But time, energy, and fatigue can certainly impact our decision making. This section explores two aspects of relational changes that affect sex as we mature and grow older: (1) our environment, and (2) our individual and relational needs.

CHANGING ENVIRONMENT AND RELATIONAL AND INDIVIDUAL NEEDS

Research reveals that the most stressful time in a marriage is when the children are teenagers. There are ongoing battles for independence. Parents incur the expense of their children's college educations. Eventually, the nest is empty. This can have a positive and a negative impact on a couple's sex life. On the positive side, there is more time to get together with greater privacy and flexibility. The negative emotional stress is the feeling of loss, especially as children become adults and launch out on their own. Parents can lose a sense of purpose and, in their grieving, lose touch with each other. If one partner is grieving and the other partner is rejoicing over the child leaving home, it may cause strife. Mothers may grieve more when a son leaves, and dads may experience a greater sense of loss when a daughter leaves.

When a child leaves for college, many stressors still can impact the marriage. Many a parent eagerly awaits "parents' weekend" at the college, only to find that it upsets the emotions again. Your child may have little time for you or they may cling to you and express many fears. Either way, as a parent you may feel helpless. Having sex with your spouse may not even be a thought you consider as your emotions run rampant, but the commitment to hold each other close can help remind you that as a couple your world is being enlarged, and your drawing close to each other offers security, strength, and companionship through the trials.

As your children grow into young adulthood they experience many of life's "hurts" that you can no longer "kiss and make better." These hurts, while technically not your own, can be emotional land mines in relationships, especially if they are internalized and not discussed or faced together. Examples may be a child failing a class, dropping out of college, losing a job, their romantic interests or lack of them, a pregnancy, or loss of a child or grandchild.

Many of us "midlifers" failed to grasp how our children's independence, or lack thereof, would impact us. At the same time, we may be adjusting to our own parents' diminished health or death. This is further complicated by our own struggles with health concerns, jobs, retirement, and preparing for changes in income.

All of these environmental factors take time and energy away from making love and from focusing on the marital relationship. Sometimes parents receive too much of their identity from parental roles and have a difficult time readjusting to being best friends and lovers. The increased time together is an adjustment all its own. The excuses for lack of intimacy and infrequent sex have to be faced head-on. A couple will need to learn to expose impasses and not be afraid of confrontation and honest discussion, even though this process may be difficult and uncomfortable. Unfortunately, because it does involve intentional choices and hard work, some couples will miss out on the benefits of working through the problems, and the deepening companionship that can result.

Midlife Issues

The forties and fifties bring many career decisions to the forefront: Will my dreams ever be realized, and will I achieve the level of success that I had hoped for? This can bring on a full-fledged midlife crisis. You may have to grieve over some of your goals and change gears.

Midlife career change and whole new career directions are common in today's marketplace. The wife may be back in the job market after full-time homemaking, and she faces many new decisions as she revs up a vocation she put on hold for the sake of mothering. The husband may be in the most productive and busiest time of his career—fighting for time to keep everything balanced and to enjoy making love.

All of that affects intimacy and a thriving sex life. The husband is entering a time when he has less sexual energy but a greater desire for intimate connecting. The wife may be entering a time of more sexual enthusiasm with greater independence and openness to explore and enjoy; or she may be experiencing the physical changes and emotional turmoil that menopause can sometimes bring. As their bodies begin to age, their circumstances are a kaleidoscope of changes and challenges. Sex can be ignored and intimacy put on the back burner, as the husband works through his challenges and the wife works at varying jobs from launching children to balancing her own career.

There will be a search for individual identity with a

need *to practice forgiveness, to negotiate competing demands, and to grieve over losses.* There can be some panic as you wonder if you have missed the perfect mate and maybe it is now or never. You may sometimes wonder what happened to the person you married. As you rediscover who your mate is, you often will desire the deeper intimacy of midlife. Don't think that you know your mate perfectly or that there are no new horizons sexually. You will want to revive mystery and plan surprises. You will not want to get into routines that cause you to neglect passionate lovemaking. It may take getting out of town (or at least out of the house) to accomplish this. Learn to nurture each other and determine as a couple to protect your relationship. It will allow you to put some pizzazz back in your love life.

Retirement Issues

The fifties and sixties face even more changes with the challenge of easing into retirement over the coming years. Retirement can be structured differently for every couple. It may be going into early retirement and a new career, or planning for more leisure time when mandatory retirement is reached and you have the challenge of filling the vacuum. Both mates can get frustrated with the husband being underfoot for the first time in their lives.

Grandparenting can bring special meaning and enjoyment; it can also bring increased demands. You may have to throw into the equation a major illness and the recuperation time involved. This is also the time in life that you start dealing with either the loss of or the increased demands of your aging parents. You may have to make difficult decisions and adjust your living situation, with a parent, child, or grandchild in your home.

Circumstances will hit the relationship with grief and losses. You may wonder if it is too late to establish a deeper level of intimacy, but you have tremendous opportunity for renewal. You are entering the years where the blessings and curses of the aging process become more apparent. Sex after fifty can become more exciting and intimate, and you can achieve a level of affirmation and togetherness as you learn to celebrate this part of your relationship. Learn your limitations and flourish within them. You know each other so well from head to foot physically. "Old dogs" can learn more tricks—be creative and experimental (see Chapter 20).

One couple had some major adjusting to do when the husband was forced into early retirement at age fifty-two. It was a financial crisis because there were still college bills to be paid for their last child, and his field did not offer an immediate lateral shift. It was also tough because they were just adjusting to their last child's leaving the nest. The wife grieved more over her empty nest than she expected but launched into a part-time job that helped fill her need for personal identity and fulfillment. Her father passed away after a struggle with cancer. It was expected but still left a hole in her life.

The husband became depressed, and the whole relationship suffered. But they rallied together. The wife grieved through her losses and started healing. They had purchased some land in the country where they were going to build a cabin and get away from the rat race.

Both found nature very therapeutic to their souls, and the cabin was a mutual goal for their sixties and seventies.

The couple valued their intimacy and worked to lessen the toll of the environment on their companionship. There were some lean times sexually due to their depression, grieving, and job fluctuations. Their marriage slowly changed—but for the better—during these times. She became more independent and he less driven, and sex came back to its place of priority.

Lovemaking became an important part of the healing. Neither minded living with ambiguity and uncertainty as much as they used to. They trusted their intimacy and could connect, separate, and reconnect more easily. Both also wanted to know they were heading toward a stable retirement and there were some things they could count on. Sex evolved into something very special in helping to meet these varied needs and staving off environmental pressures. They entered into a very intimate time—a second, or maybe a third or fourth honeymoon.

Later Life Losses

As a couple moves into their seventies and eighties, they are well into retirement and facing the fact of losing each other eventually as health deteriorates. It is a time when suffering can build character as you transcend yourself and let go of control. This is more than a philosophical concept. It becomes *your* reality. You may have to fight through some new boundaries as you set up ground rules around leisure routines and chores. Don't isolate or become too dependent.

Sexually, the older body will creak and groan, but

don't let inertia set in. Continue to enjoy sexual closeness even if it doesn't frequently include intercourse—though it may. Eric Erickson, in his research in sexuality at various stages of the life cycle, found that older people experience a more generalized form of sexuality, as opposed to specific sexuality. This means that they may become more sensuous while having intercourse less often.[1] Fight for your privacy if you are living with your children and enjoy the fruit of many years of bonding and sharing. Say nice things to each other, and hold each other close. You will start to fear losing each other, and it will be okay to desperately clutch the other one close now and again. Sex can have a transcendent beauty that is admirable for a younger couple to emulate. The following anecdote reflects the importance of a humorous and healthy attitude about later life.

Two retired people, Jacob, age ninety-two, and Harriet, age eighty-nine, are all excited about their decision to get married. They go for a stroll to discuss the wedding, and on the way they pass a drugstore. Jacob suggests they go in. Jacob addresses the man behind the counter: "Are you the owner?" The pharmacist answers, "Yes," and the conversation continues as follows:

> Jacob: "We're about to get married. Do you sell
>   heart medication?"
> Pharmacist: "Of course we do."
> Jacob: "How about medicine for circulation?"
> Pharmacist: "All kinds."
> Jacob: "Medicine for rheumatism, scoliosis?"
> Pharmacist: "Definitely."

Jacob: "How about V-i-a-g-r-a—?"

Pharmacist: "Of course."

Jacob: "Medicine for memory problems, arthritis, jaundice?"

Pharmacist: "Yes, a large variety. The works."

Jacob: "What about vitamins, sleeping pills, Geritol, antidotes for Parkinson's disease?"

Pharmacist: "Absolutely."

Jacob: "You sell wheelchairs and walkers?"

Pharmacist: "All speeds and sizes."

Jacob: "We'd like to use this store as our Bridal Registry."

In a survey of older adults by Tim and Beverly LaHaye, they found that "40 percent of couples are doing practically nothing to keep the romantic fires burning."[2] As we get older and move through the "labyrinth of life," it becomes more critical than ever that we "gear up" romantically so we can find comfort and security in the intimacy we share as a couple. This may be an excellent time to pull out your marriage vows and rewrite them in a way that reflects your commitment to each other in your own individualized circumstances. Life has a much broader perspective now. And while the "new" may be worn off the initial romantic relationship, a deeper and more fulfilling relationship can take its place—one that includes romance, adventure, and surprise, but all of it seen through the eyes of experience and a deep care that will carry you through to the end.

Chapter 8

When It Isn't Working: *Male and Female Sexual Challenges*

*H*ere's the bad news: Both men and women will struggle with a variety of sexual difficulties throughout their lives, and some sexual dysfunctions will tend to increase as we get older. Nobody likes this, but the good news is that medical and psychological solutions exist to help resolve these challenges. More good news occurs as a couple confronts their challenges together, and in a supportive and nurturing way, work to find solutions. Facing the adversity in this manner will result in an enhanced relationship.

Both sexes may have to contend with difficulties in desire, arousal, and orgasm. For men, these concerns may revolve around erectile dysfunction and delayed ejaculation. For women, there can be problems with painful intercourse and hormonal changes. We devote Chapter 12 to dealing with the lack of sexual desire, and Chapter 4 addressed the hormonal concerns related to menopause.

Sexual responses and malfunctions can be very complex. This chapter will not be exhaustive, but it can be a starting point as you press through to finding the resources you need to work out the problem. Your sexual difficulty may be partly or primarily a physical or medical problem. This will require the assistance of a medical professional who can diagnose and treat. Many other factors may be contributing to your problems. Your relationship with your spouse has a significant impact on your sexual enjoyment. In other words, my sexual responsiveness and problems affect his/her responsiveness. If she is having pain in intercourse, husbands don't want to hurt their mates and will back off or lose erections.

Are you exhausted, depressed, under stress, or tremendously focused on your job? All these conditions impact your ability to feel and be sexual. Some personality styles create a propensity for sexual dysfunction. The worrier who is sensitive to environmental stress and anxiety will be more prone to performance anxiety. Attention deficit and obsessive-compulsive disorders can contribute to thinking and behaviors that help prolong impotence or delayed ejaculation.

SEEK MEDICAL INTERVENTION

In treating any sexual malfunction, ruling out and treating any physical problems is the place to start. Get a thorough physical to check things like blood pressure, testosterone, estrogen, thyroid, and prostate. With complications like ED (erectile dysfunction), you may need to find a urologist who specializes in sexual problems. Medical science has grown in its ability to diagnose blood flow and nerve problems, and surgical alternatives have dramatically improved.

BE OPEN TO COUNSELING

There are times when a marriage therapist can help with relational problems that may be interfering with your sex life. You may need a counselor with skill in sexual issues or a trained sex therapist to help diagnose and coach you through the sexual challenges. They can provide self-help exercises that can be utilized to overcome your problem.

DISEASES AND MEDICATION COMPLICATIONS

Start with the physical and then proceed to the psychological. If you are battling diabetes, working on your relationship with your spouse will help, but you will need to understand the effects of the disease first. Conversely, just dealing with the medical and healing the physical will not put you in a place to want to make love to your partner. Chapter 9 addresses many of the diseases or disabilities that can interfere with sexual function, and Chapter 10 looks at the effects of medications on the process. Again, check with your doctor regarding any use of antidepressants, antihypertensives for high blood pressure, and some ulcer medications. Sometimes adjusting the dosage, switching the drug, or adding another agent can help, or depending on the medication, a brief day vacation from the medication can help sexual functioning.

AROUSAL DIFFICULTIES

In women, difficulty with arousal before or during intercourse involves the inability to attain or maintain adequate genital lubrication, swelling or other physical response, such as nipple sensitivity, or sensitivity of the clitoris or labia. Arousal problems may result from emotional stress, such as depression or ongoing marital tension, a lack of sufficient stimulation, or a physical problem, such as diminished blood flow to the vagina or clitoris.

Initially, women experiencing low or no arousal with vaginal dryness should try using commercial lubricants or vitamin E oils or mineral oils when they engage in sex. Inadequate stimulation contributes to arousal disorders, especially in older women, and may be helped by taking more time to touch each other and fondle, or using a vibrator to increase stimulation. Often women who develop arousal problems are thinking negative thoughts about themselves or their partner while they are making love. (Most women are not even aware they are doing this negative thinking until they are given the assignment to "listen" to themselves the next time they are sexually involved with their spouse.) Negative thinking *is* a turnoff.

Taking a warm bath before intercourse can help a woman to relax and also may increase arousal. Check your body and your mind for anxiety and distractions. When the vagina and penis do not respond to our expectations, anxiety is created. And with anxiety can come frustration, which can be inappropriately vented on your mate. Remember, it can be as uncaring to say to a woman, "Get some (artificial) lubrication," as for her to say, "Why don't you go and get a prosthesis for your penis." Anxiety inhibits arousal, so exploring and learning anxiety-reduction techniques (deep breaths and making choices in what to focus on) can be helpful. Though not an easy task, arousal is dependent on keeping your body, mind, and heart truly present in your lovemaking.

Erectile Dysfunction (ED)

By the age of forty, around 90 percent of men have experienced one or more times of having difficulty getting or sustaining an erection. It still surprises most couples when it occurs, and this is often followed by an overreaction by both mates. This malfunction is prone to being made worse by anxiety and frustrated reactions.

Understanding ED. Erectile problems can be caused by physical or psychological problems, or a combination of both. A total lack of erection or a lack of firmness in the erection could point to physical problems. As we discussed in Chapter 5, the process of aging makes erections more difficult to achieve without direct physical stimulation, and they may slightly decrease in firmness. The presence of nighttime/morning erections or the ability to get erections in self-stimulation would point to psychological causes.

The most common psychological cause of ED is performance anxiety. Getting sexually aroused and getting an erection depend on the autonomic nervous system. A man doesn't will an erection to occur—it happens as he is stimulated, physically and emotionally, into arousal. These reflexive nerve responses are short-circuited by anxiety. Psychological impotence is usually not the first time an erection does not occur. It happens with the subsequent fear of not getting or losing an erection.

It's Friday night and the husband is exhausted and has had too much to drink. He cannot get an erection. Saturday morning he fearfully tries to make love again. He, and sometimes his wife, are no longer present; they are mentally up on the bedpost as spectators, wondering if he will get an erection this time. This performance anxiety becomes the kiss of death to enjoying lovemaking.

Various forms of stress can also decrease your ability to focus on sexual feelings and become sufficiently stimulated. Environmental stressors can produce an inhibiting feeling such as *depression*, which is a common cause of sexual problems. You will want to discuss with your doctor whether it might be a factor in your life. *Grief* is another emotion that can be a real sexual depressant and create less desire and an inability to become aroused. *Relationships* also have an important impact on your sex life. It may be the depression and grief of your close relationships that are creating the loss and hurt. It is a myth that men are never affected by their emotions and always have a strong libido.

Certain physical problems can interfere with getting erections. Hormones trigger desire, and the autonomic nervous system sends a signal causing the penis to engorge with blood and become erect. Diseases like diabetes, multiple sclerosis, and kidney problems can interfere with the nervous system and its functioning. Some surgeries like prostatectomy (removing the prostate) may destroy nerve paths. Radiation treatment can affect nerves and blood supply, creating leakage from the penis.

Medical Interventions in ED. An insufficient level of the hormone testosterone can create lack of desire and difficulty functioning. Hormone deficiency can be checked out with a simple blood test to assess one's testosterone level and also luteinizing hormone (LH) levels. LH levels are necessary to assess whether a person may have pituitary or hypothalamus deficits or even testicular failure. Once this assessment is completed, the physician can determine whether testosterone replacement is appropriate.

Remember that testosterone replacement is clinically effective for the improvement of desire or sex drive in low-testosterone males. It is not particularly effective in restoring erections. Drugs can also interfere with sexual functioning. For more information about medication effects, refer to Chapter 10.

The most common treatment for ED are the PDE5 inhibitors (e.g., Viagra, Levitra, Cialis), with a success rate of about 70 percent. These medications have the effect of widening the blood vessels in the penis. They only will work, however, in the context of desire and physical stimulation. They are not to be given to men taking nitrate drugs (like nitroglycerin), often used to control chest pain, because they increase the possibility of a dramatic drop in blood pressure.[1]

If the PDE5 inhibitors don't work physiologically, consult a urologist. Other drugs such as apomorphine or phentolamine, administered orally or under the tongue, may be tried that deal with other parts of the body and central nervous system. Sometimes chemical injections that can be self-administered (prostaglandin E, phentolomine, or papaverine) are other proven means of treating ED. Prostagladin E (Alprostadil) also comes in a pellet form that can be inserted into the urethra, which then dissolves into the blood stream. The injections should not be utilized with men with certain blood diseases like sickle cell anemia. If the erection does not subside after four to six hours, this is called priapism. Seek medical help immediately or you may risk the possibility of permanent impotence.[2]

There is also a vacuum pump that your physician can prescribe to pull blood into the penis, with a ring to maintain the erection. It is interesting that some of the nuisance of self-injections or the vacuum pump make them more difficult for people to follow through with these interventions. Newer surgical techniques have been perfected to deal with blood flow and nerve damage. A urologist who specializes in sexual dysfunction can help diagnose whether these surgical interventions are feasible.

A physician can also help in sorting through the advisability of a penile prosthesis after truly determining that the impotence is indeed physiological and permanent. The most commonly used prosthesis is inflatable (a second is a semirigid rod) and is inserted in the penis with a pump mechanism in the scrotum. Psychological counseling can help sort through both mates' feelings and sexual needs. Erectile dysfunction does not prevent a man from having orgasms and ejaculating, and some couples adjust to the impossibility of having intercourse. They emphasize other aspects of making love and feel content and close. Others find a prosthesis revolutionizes their sex lives.

An important part of dealing with ED is heading it off before it becomes a chronic dilemma. Eating a low-fat diet and exercising regularly can help dramatically. Men with waistlines of forty-two inches or greater are 200 percent more likely to experience sexual dysfunction. Men who do not exercise are 50 percent more likely to have dysfunction than men who exercise twenty to thirty minutes daily. If you smoke, stop! One study found that men who smoked a pack a day for twenty years had a 60 percent greater chance of becoming impotent than did nonsmokers.[3]

Couples can wisely and lovingly handle some of the psychological issues and prevent an occurrence of impotence from evolving into a recurrent problem. *The wife has an important role* in taking incidents of ED in stride and not panicking. She can emphasize that ED is normal in all men. She can help both forget about trying to have sex immediately and wait until another time when they are rested and able to focus on pleasure. Minimizing the incident is the best medicine. Caress, play, and enjoy each other as you take the focus off intercourse! This is not a commentary on your skill or attractiveness as a lover. Learn when to initiate and when to refuse so you don't attempt sex when you are not in the mood.

ORGASM DIFFICULTIES

An orgasm is an intense sensation occurring at the peak of sexual arousal and followed by release of sexual tension.

In women, an orgasm is a series of rhythmic muscular contractions of the vagina and uterus accompanied by sharp increases in pulse rate, blood pressure, and breathing rate, and muscle contractions throughout the body.

Some women have never experienced an orgasm. This time of life creates time and energy for becoming orgasmic. Helpful resources exist that can assist in this journey.[4]

Others become distressed because their orgasm is less intense than in the past, or is delayed. Less intensity or an occasional lack of orgasm may be a natural product of aging. Don't panic; this may be an incident and not a habit. The most common cause of lack of orgasm is insufficient stimulation and arousal. The inability to be orgasmic can also be caused by emotional trauma, sexual abuse, hormone deficiency, and insufficient blood flow or damage to the pelvic nerves due to surgery. Some medications like antidepressants can slow down the orgasmic response. It can also be inhibited by stored-up resentments against your spouse.

Delayed Ejaculation

Delayed (sometimes called inhibited) ejaculation is less common than premature ejaculation and impotence. It is most easily defined as any time the husband cannot reach a climax as quickly as he desires. Some of the common causes of delayed ejaculation vary, depending on the situation. One man experienced stress and anxiety about a variety of midlife experiences. His wife, with her own stressors, was not as active in the lovemaking process. All combined to lessen his sexual focus and arousal.

The husband sometimes finds the vagina too loose or

too lubricated to give sufficient friction. If that is so, the wife can practice Kegel exercises and tighten the muscles of her vaginal opening. She may wish to consult a gynecologist or a cosmetic surgeon to tighten the vagina if Kegel exercises don't improve friction. Proceed with caution. It might not be the vagina at all but a lack of sexual arousal and focused concentration on the husband's part. The ability to focus on growing sexual arousal is a crucial part of great sex.

Sometimes emotional scars, family repression, or sexual guilt or intimidation interfere with a man's ability to experience pleasure with intercourse. Often the husband can climax with manual stimulation but through intercourse only with difficulty. Stopping masturbating and allowing the sensations of penis in vagina (very different from a hand) to grow erotically arousing may help.

Delayed ejaculation can also be drug-induced. Chapter 10 addresses the effects of medications on sexual function. You should attempt to have an open discussion with your doctor about the nature of the medications you are taking and the risks of sexual dysfunction accordingly. Inform your physician of any side effects you may be experiencing, so that it may be specifically addressed at each visit and adjustments can be made.

PAINFUL INTERCOURSE

Dyspareunia involves recurrent or persistent genital pain associated with sexual intercourse. It can develop due to vaginal infections, thinning of the vaginal lining during menopause, bladder or urethral infection, pelvic inflammatory disease, endometriosis, some vaginal or vulval surgical procedures, as well as various psychological issues or relationship problems.

Lowered estrogen over a period of months causes the vaginal lining to become thin and dry (as it does during menopause); therefore, intercourse hurts. We cannot stress enough: When sex is painful, emotionally or physically, DO NOT "PLAY THROUGH THE PAIN." Get help! Painful sex does not get better by ignoring it or trying to play through it. Often, it further traumatizes and creates more sexual difficulties.

As we discussed in Chapter 4, during menopause, most women experience sexual changes due to hormonal shifts. Muscle tone in the vagina declines, and the muscles don't contract as easily (or not at all). Up to 40 percent of menopausal women develop dyspareunia if they do not use some type of estrogen replacement.

Treating Painful Intercourse

Keep on hand plenty of artificial lubricant. This is sold in most pharmacies and even in grocery stores, in a gel or a more liquid form. You can also use natural oils, from coconut or almond to olive oil. These are edible and don't interfere with oral stimulation of the genitals. They also may be appealing for scent or consistency. Vegetable oils (corn or safflower) work fine if you have forgotten to purchase other artificial lubrication. The advantage of artificial lubricants is they are often water soluble and easier for the vagina to self-cleanse. Use lubricants generously when the vagina is irritated or there is anxiety. It is amazing how much pain can be prevented by using common sense!

Gentle and *slow* are crucial words in overcoming painful intercourse. Creating a safe and tender atmosphere is important in dealing with stress and tension. Unwind together. Work on relaxing and being playful. Allow the wife to set the pace. Allow plenty of time for love play and arousal before attempting intercourse. Try using a position (such as wife on top) that lets her control penetration and depth. Take your time and enjoy the process. Be imaginative in creating ambience.

Stop when there is pain! Shift your position. Stop thrusting, or stop deep thrusting. Prop a small pillow underneath the hips or lower back, use more lubrication, or go back to loving, playful caressing. Relax again. Use your creativity, but *never* ignore the discomfort. If no immediate intervention helps, stop making love and just hold each other, or bring each other to orgasm in other ways until the problem can be checked out medically.

Sexual challenges are not catastrophes. They can be overcome. Other skills can be helpful as you and your mate work through these issues. Learn to communicate effectively and build a loving companionship that is full of playfulness, honesty, and erotic tension.

Chapter 9

Loving Through the Obstacles:
Dealing with Disease and Disability

Even though we would prefer not to believe it, disease and disabilities are inevitable for most aging couples. Even relatively healthy people occasionally will suffer from illness or disabling circumstances. They may take the form of brief or chronic illnesses, or short- or long-term disabilities. Periodic health problems are a given with aging, but how we handle these challenges is not so fixed. At times our traditional ways of making love may be a part of the fallout, but positive, sensual lovemaking can still be a healthy part of our lives.

A committed, loving relationship is the most important part of making love, and relationships can actually deepen and grow as couples learn to cope with challenges. The purpose of this chapter is to address a variety of the physical obstacles that often impact couples after midlife and provide specific strategies so that we can learn to love beyond the obstacles and discover a place of greater wholeness. The message is that we can make positive changes in our lovemaking by learning new skills, building erotic fantasy, and modifying our own warm, unique, and exciting lovemaking together.

There are many chronic illnesses as well as some disabilities (and/or their treatments) that can interfere with sexual functioning. These difficulties may affect sexuality in either direct or indirect ways. Let's discuss several medical problems and their impact on sexual function.

DIABETES

Because of nerve and vascular damage, a man with diabetes may have problems getting and maintaining adequate erections for intercourse. Impotence is often the first sign of the disease. However, nearly half of all diabetic men suffer impotence for psychological reasons due to erectile difficulties early in the disease that leave them anxious, feeling inadequate, and fearful of more failures.[1] To minimize psychological anxiety, a man and his wife may go to other activities in their lovemaking and not make erections and intercourse the be-all and end-all. In women, diabetes can make it more difficult to achieve arousal and orgasm due to a loss of sensation in the genitals and vaginal dryness. Diabetes often leads to lower estrogen levels and can intensify the hormonal impact during menopause, so a woman should ask her physician if she is a good candidate for estrogen replacement therapy.

It is important to note that the sexual impact of diabetes can often be minimized if one rigorously follows the prescribed medical and dietary regimens. The various impotence treatments mentioned in Chapter 8 might prove helpful in diabetic men. Talk to your doctor regarding your options or talk to a sex therapist if you need help overcoming the psychological effects of impotence.

ARTHRITIS

Arthritis is a common chronic illness that causes pain and stiffening of affected joints. Loosening arthritic joints and stiff backs before making love helps. Heating pads and warm baths can be helpful and even sensual; shared, they can become a part of love play. The couple can associate pain-relieving rubs with erotic arousal—do make sure you wash medicated creams off your hands prior to touching your spouse's genitals. Taking pain medications or anti-inflammatory agents before love play may also allow for windows of time with decreased pain. During those times, couples will find it easier to focus and enjoy each other sexually. If the pain medication seems to decrease sexual interest, arousal, and/or the ability to attain an orgasm, talk to your doctor about changing the prescription or lowering the dose.

During love play, it is often helpful to support arthritic joints with pillows and to avoid positions that put stress on joints. For example, the husband could sit propped against the headboard of the bed with pillows and a heating pad on his lower back. The wife could then sit between his legs with her back against him or lie back with her genital area in his lap. These positions allow for mutual pleasure with less wear on bodies. Practice positions of intercourse that allow you to lie down and stay less active. Crosswise positions and certain rear-entry positions may be easier. Substituting a side-by-side position for the on-top position may help aching knees and allow active participation (see Chapter 18). If arthritic hands make manual stimulation uncomfortable, oral stimulation may be a good alternative.

Monitor what works for you and your partner, and research your disease to learn about what moves and positions will or won't increase pain in the partner with arthritis. If you have experienced joint replacement surgery, you should be able to resume sexual activity six weeks after surgery. Individuals who undergo hip replacement surgery will need to work with their physical therapist and physician regarding what sexual positions will prevent dislocation of their new joint.

HEART DISEASE

Heart disease, heart attack, and heart surgery often result in individuals and their partners being concerned that resuming sexual activity will result in a worsening of the heart condition or sudden death. Yet, less than 1 percent of heart attack fatalities occur during sexual activity, and most individuals can safely resume their lovemaking.[2] Couples are encouraged to resume their activity slowly and not to expect too much too soon. Additionally, since there is an indication that increased stress predisposes individuals to further problems, couples are cautioned when resuming sexual activity to stick with familiar routines and places. Since the major effect of a heart attack on sexuality is psychological, you may need to be reassured by your physician that it is safe to resume lovemaking. The emotional benefits of lovemaking usually outweigh the physical risk. If angina pains are troubling or unpredictable, or you experience shortness of breath, check with your doctor about the possibility of taking a nitroglycerine tablet before beginning lovemaking. Be sure to avoid the use of Viagra-like drugs if you do use nitroglycerine.

CANCER

The psychological effect of a cancer diagnosis and the discomfort of treatment can have particularly devastating consequences on making love. Most cancer diagnoses affect both partners. It is beneficial to learn about the cancer, its treatments, the healing process, and the possible impact of the cancer and treatment on sexuality. Just facing the possibility of death with ensuing panic, grief, and depression affects sexuality. The body-image dragon may rear its ugly head with surgeries, especially a mastectomy. The cancer survivor and his/her spouse may need to restructure their attitudes as they discover new and exciting ways of arousal and sexual enjoyment.

Cancer treatments are linked to low sexual desire, erection problems, difficulty reaching orgasm, dry or weaker orgasm, and infertility.[3] Cancer surgery and treatment can sometimes damage nerves, which may lead to erectile or lubrication problems. Sometimes radiation and chemotherapy may affect sexual desire or physical arousal and lubrication over a period of months, until nerves and tissue can be regenerated. Severe fatigue is a common problem during and following cancer treatment, necessitating a reduction or elimination of once-enjoyed activities.

Treatment for colorectal cancer can result in unpredictable smells and accidents. These smells and accidents can be minimized by planning sexual activities when your colostomy is not active and avoiding foods that produce gas. Cancer treatment also impacts body image because people may experience disfigurement from surgeries, lose weight, lose muscle mass, or lose their hair, including pubic and facial hair. It's not unusual for a person undergoing radical cancer treatment to suffer periods of body loathing.

Remember, in the early stages of treatment the issue is not about sex, but survival. Intimacy is more than just intercourse, and the nondisabled spouse's flexibility with roles, willingness to participate in care, and support and encouragement will prove essential to the healing process. It is important to discuss fears and desires prior to resuming sexual activity following or during treatment for cancer. Go gently when viewing and touching a mutilated body part for the first time. Many individuals undergoing treatment for cancer appreciate being held gently and tenderly by their partners. Soft, tender words, combined with gentle stroking, can convey caring, support, and love. Allow yourself and your partner time to grieve.

Prostate Cancer

It has been said that every man will contract prostate cancer if he lives long enough. The good news is that new available treatments such as nerve-sparing surgical techniques as well as radiation therapy have led to fewer problems for those being treated for prostate cancer. However, even with the "nerve-sparing" procedures, it can be several months before erectile function is regained and intercourse is possible. Often, medications like Viagra are prescribed soon after surgery to encourage genital blood flow even when erection is not yet possible. The man is also encouraged to manually stimulate his penis in order to regain erectile function. This can be a rehabilitative "exercise" that the couple can enjoy together. It is important to be very patient during this process, as it is often months before function is regained. Depending on the treatment, men may experience considerable variation in the quality of their orgasm and ejaculation. Sometimes the sphincter does not close off and the ejaculate goes back into the bladder with the orgasm (retrograde ejaculation). When nerves are damaged during a prostatectomy and permanent impotency results, there are implant options available. Please refer to Chapter 8 for a more thorough discussion.

HYSTERECTOMY

Hysterectomy is the surgical removal of a woman's uterus and is a common treatment for excessive bleeding, fibroid tumors, and endometriosis. The good news about menopause is that many women who are plagued with fibroid tumors and endometriosis find that when their periods stop, their tumors shrink and their endometriosis comes to an end. To prevent unnecessary hysterectomies, women are encouraged to obtain second medical opinions. In fact, many insurance companies now require second opinions for this common surgery. Hysterectomies may result in a change in genital sensations, arousal, and orgasm as well as being psychologically traumatic for some women, especially if they associate their worth as women to the uterus. However, it is false that a hysterectomy causes weight gain, prohibits sexual functioning, or accelerates the aging process.

Hormone replacement therapy may be prescribed (especially if a woman's ovaries were also removed). The couple may find vaginal dryness an issue after hysterectomy and may want to try some of the vaginal lubricants suggested in Chapters 3 and 8. The husband's support and understanding are vitally important, and he should learn about the sexual side effects of the surgery and of HRT, assure her of her desirability through comments and affection, and not pressure her for sex before she is ready.

STROKE

Strokes may impact a person's ability to move and feel touch on one side of their body. Along with these physical changes, stroke victims may have a depressed or quickly changeable mood, speech and comprehension problems, and altered memory and thinking processes. Many stroke survivors need assistance in taking care of their hygiene needs. These changes can spill over into the sexual realm, creating anxiety and performance concerns.[4] Erotic massage to the unaffected body areas can be very arousing since the stroke victim may develop heightened sensitivity in the areas not damaged by the stroke. Sexual activity should be reintroduced slowly by touching and caressing. Memory loss can affect sexual functioning if a partner has forgotten some aspects of lovemaking. It is important to initiate sex when both are rested and before a meal (to reduce strain on the heart).

The following suggestions are included to help individuals with urinary catheters be sexual: Males are encouraged to fold the catheter back over the erect penis and place a lubricated condom over the catheter and penis. Females are encouraged to tape the catheter to their abdomen or thigh and to use an adequate water-soluble lubricant. Strokes may negatively impact balance and as a result, couples may want to use a side-lying position with the paralyzed limbs supported with pillows. Be creative as you experiment with different positions.

CHRONIC PAIN

Chronic pain hits young and old. It may be an old sports injury, back problems, a knee or hip replacement, severe arthritis, or nerve damage from mastectomy or other cancer surgery. Sex may be the furthest thing from a person's mind when the pain is intense. For some, making love or an orgasm may intensify the pain, and for others it can be a relief and distraction. Unfortunately, some pain medications can negatively affect sexual desire and ability to achieve orgasm and may need to be adjusted if possible.

With many types of chronic pain, if you wait till it feels okay—you will never make love. It helps to increase your communication with your spouse about what is pleasurable and minimizes your pain. You may have a difficult time tuning out the winces and grimaces of pain and not losing arousal. With practice at hitting the optimal times and knowing when to adjust or even stop love play, sexual frequency increases. Often the mate without the pain needs to initiate and encourage their spouse with pillows and props and some seduction. But the person who has the pain needs to "call the shots" and communicate what they can and cannot do, and this should be respected and honored. Positions that allow the spouse who is experiencing pain to control movement during intercourse will be important. Remember that muscle-stretching exercises and hot baths may also be helpful before lovemaking.

SURGERIES

Following many surgical procedures, a period of abstinence from intercourse may be necessary for several weeks or even months to allow adequate time for recovery. Often, individuals may experience postoperative depression that can dampen desire and may require time for support, communication, and encouragement. Loving touch can be very helpful in encouraging intimacy and in nurturing the relationship during the recovery period. Be sure to talk to your doctor about how and when to resume sexual activity.

SIX NECESSARY SKILLS

Illnesses and disabilities present different challenges in roles and attitudes to males and females. But there is much commonality in working through such a challenge to a fulfilling sex life. Certain skills make a difference if learned and employed consistently. This section discusses six of them.

1. Creating a Positive Sexual Self-Image

Everyone struggles at times with body image and the comfortable enjoyment of masculinity or femininity. This can be especially true of an illness or disability. However, it is an exciting phenomenon that we have the ability to become what we think we are. Our attitudes and beliefs about ourselves are crucial. It may help to read Chapter 6 on body image and rediscovering attractiveness.

2. Communicating

If you want to live as a comfortable friend and lover, learn to communicate with your spouse about the loss of personal control and many other emotionally loaded topics. Certain illnesses and disabilities require you to rely on others when dealing with bodily wastes, and control over bodily functions is often taken out of your hands and made a public matter. Talk to your mate. Become excellent sounding boards for each other. Learn how to dialogue. Read Chapter 13 on communicating sexually.

3. Developing Flexibility

Take the time and energy to talk about the structure of your sex life. Provide courage and romantic creativity for each other as you find different ways to make love. Talk through possible ways to adapt sexual foreplay and positions that overcome limitations.

4. Expanding Your Senses and Knowledge of Sexuality

We each have a body and mind that God created to enjoy pleasure, but we use only about one-third of their full sensual capacity. Individuals and couples need to more fully allow their bodies to take in sensual pleasure—which so easily spills over into their sexual lives. Enjoy using all five of your senses. We are still learning how the brain takes in and stores data. It is exciting how when one sense is disabled, another expands. The person who is blind develops a keener sense of hearing and touch. Different sexual behaviors and parts of the body can take on new meaning—creating a warm closeness or exciting arousal.

5. Choosing Optimal Times

Ask specific sexual questions of your medical doctor about what is permitted physically and what is not. Ask for and find pamphlets on your particular disability. Be an informed lover and determine what physical sensations and types of sexual activity are possible as you maximize lovemaking.

Prioritizing your activities is important. The energy to do what you used to do probably won't be there. Face important difficult questions: What can I let go of? What do I want to save energy for today? Quality lovemaking will depend on your planning.

6. Grieving

Elisabeth Kübler-Ross and other psychological researchers have demonstrated that people go through various stages and feelings when they are grieving a loss

(shock, denial, anger, bargaining, depression, and acceptance). You and your partner may have experienced multiple losses: the marriage as it was, autonomy, dreams and
expectations, sexual self-image, and mutual health—to
name a few. The one-flesh companionship has been
shaken up in many ways, and the sexual part may be
most obvious. Grieve these losses personally and together.

THE NONDISABLED PARTNER

The feelings of the nondisabled or non-ill partner will
range all over the map, much as those of the partner with
the disability—from despair to optimism (sometimes
false around a possible cure), from anger and discourage-
ment to joy and pleasure. Sometimes it may be difficult
to switch from the role of helping your disabled mate to
being a passionate lover.

As the nondisabled partner, you will probably have to
assume a more active behavioral (not emotional) role to
encourage sensuality. You may be asked to do things like
deal with bowel or bladder accidents or perhaps try
types of oral stimulation that you might have found
unpleasant in the past. New behaviors will be required
as you and your mate pleasure each other. Learning new
and effective lovemaking techniques is seldom comfortable or smooth, whether you are disabled or not. It may
be helpful to talk to a counselor or an occupational or
physical therapist regarding any problems. However,
don't treat your partner as fragile. You need to process
your feelings, too, as you work through to practical solutions in your lovemaking.

Stay creative and pray for extra strength. Your stamina and hope will be needed, especially if your mate is adjusting to a recent disability that has impacted their self-image. Create an effective support network as you affirm your sexual partnership. Marital trauma and divorce can occur because of lack of knowledge. Just because your spouse may look better or you wish your spouse felt better doesn't necessarily mean that the situation has changed. Keep seeking information and courageously face reality.

Disability can be a time of discovery about making love and building a better sexual relationship. Couples can build stronger love and intimacy through the hardship. Timing, taking initiative, following medical advice, and separating being nurse from being lover are important. Creatively seek solutions to new obstacles as you patiently and proactively talk for hours. Lean on others for hope, encouragement, and help. Push professionals for better answers. God will bless you on this journey. *Remember:* How we respond to the obstacles in our lives often determines the degree of intimacy in our love life when we're beyond the obstacle.

Chapter 10

Medication Busters and Boosters:
How Drugs Affect Sex

row of bottles on my shelf caused me
   to analyze myself.
One yellow pill I hope to pop goes to my heart
   so it won't stop.
A little white one that I take, goes to my hands
   so they won't shake.
The blue ones that I use a lot, tell me I'm happy
   when I'm not.
The purple pill goes to my brain, and tells me
   that I have no pain.
The capsules tell me not to sneeze, or cough, or
   choke or even wheeze.
The red ones, smallest of them all, go to my blood
   so I won't fall.

The orange ones so big and bright, stop my leg
    cramps in the night.
Such an array of brilliant pills helping to cure
    all kinds of ills.
But what I'd really like to know, is what tells
    each one where to go.

                      (Author unknown)

Perhaps you can relate to this poem that describes the experience of many as the prevalence of medication increases as we age. And, *all drugs have side effects.*

Many times it may be the medication—not disease, disability, psychological or relational concerns that can cause a sexual problem. As we grow older, the likelihood is that we will be taking multiple medications. At midlife, medications are often prescribed to lower blood pressure, regulate heart conditions, treat depression, control ulcers, and treat a variety of aches, pains, colds, and allergies. More than two hundred commonly prescribed medications can influence sexual function or enjoyment. The most common sexual side effects include decreased libido, impotence or difficulty getting or maintaining an erection, loss of sensation in the genitals, increased vaginal dryness, or a difficulty with ejaculation in men or orgasm in women.

The human body with its blood vessels, nerves, hormones, and brain chemistry is wonderfully complex. This chapter will especially consider biochemistry and medications that can negatively affect sexual desire in our bodies. It is important to remember that most illnesses, especially chronic illness, take a real toll on sexual desire too.

It is interesting that all medications and drugs have

side effects, and many have sexual side effects in varying degrees. Alcohol is a depressant, while a common cold remedy like an antihistamine dries out our sinus passages and the female vagina. People are encouraged to talk to their physicians and pharmacists about the possible sexual side effects of the prescription and over-the-counter medications they take. If you don't ask, they often will not tell you about the potential for sexual side effects.

In trying to understand the effects of drugs on the sexual process, let's take a look at a simplified explanation that describes how this mechanism functions in our bodies.

The brain is our most important sexual organ, and sexual activity is initiated and controlled in the brain by a number of chemical messengers (neurotransmitters, peptides, and hormones) that communicate through nerve cells called neurons. Neurons have thousands of receptors to receive the chemical messages, much like a lock would receive a key. As a neurotransmitter fits into its specific receptor, a series of actions occurs and the body will respond accordingly. Some of these neurotransmitters encourage excitatory responses (often favorable for sexual function), and some will result in inhibitory actions (may be unfavorable for sexual function).

There are dozens of neurotransmitters, many of which we know very little about, but three types of neurotransmitters are very influential in our sexual physiology—norepinephrine, dopamine, and serotonin.

Norepinephrine is the key chemical in general physical and mental arousal. It works like a battery current that must be activated in order for the rest of the sexual mechanism to ignite and operate. Norepinephrine stimulates desire and arousal in that it produces an alerting, focusing, orienting response (similar to the fight or flight response), as well as regulating blood pressure. However, this kind of stimulation causes a constriction of some blood vessels and can interfere with getting and keeping an erection. Basic behaviors like hunger, thirst, and emotion, as well as sex, may be caused by norepinephrine release.

Dopamine is the pleasure chemical in the brain and is the primary neurotransmitter involved in sex drive, attraction, desire, arousal, response, orgasm, and satisfaction. It makes us feel good. This may be why cocaine and amphetamines are so addicting and pleasurable in that these drugs stimulate dopamine receptors. An alteration in dopamine accounts for two major disorders. Too much dopamine activation results in the psychotic condition of schizophrenia. Too little dopamine activation can result in Parkinson's disease.

Serotonin functions to prevent excessive excitation and decrease anxiety and aggressiveness. It helps to regulate mood as well as functioning in sleep, wakefulness, temperature regulation, and feeding behaviors. It helps make people nicer and functions as a balance to norepinephrine and dopamine. However, in so doing, it can inhibit arousal and orgasm.

Arousal begins when the dopamine-activated brain sends a message to the genitals that sexual activity is possible. Norepinephrine is involved in this nerve transmission down the spinal cord to the pelvic area and genitals. Serotonin plays a role in helping people be nice to each other so that sex may be possible and in controlling the sexual urges so that the sex is not aberrant or overly aggressive.

The sex hormones (e.g., estrogen, progesterone, and

testosterone) have a profound influence on the neuro-transmitter actions that mediate sexual behavior, and account for the intricate ups and downs of sexual arousal, functioning, and pleasure.[1] Dopamine and testosterone are symbiotic in that they tend to stimulate each other's release. Serotonin and estrogen also function in a similar manner with each other. A proper balance in the brain and body of these and other neurotransmitters and hormones is necessary for desire, arousal, and orgasm to occur, and anything that interrupts the cascade of signals and reflexes in neurotransmission can cause sexual dysfunction.

SEXUAL BUSTERS

Medications can serve as sex busters or boosters, depending on the type of impact they have on neurotransmitters and hormones. The commonly prescribed medications and drugs of abuse that can cause difficulties in sexual functioning include, but are not limited to, testosterone-lowering drugs, heart medications, anticancer agents, antihistamines, blood pressure medications, hormones (e.g., corticosteroids, progestins), illicit and nonprescription drugs (e.g., alcohol, cocaine, nicotine, amphetamines, marijuana), painkillers (e.g., Demerol, Methadone), and psychiatric medications (e.g., drugs to treat depression, ADHD, anxiety, bipolar disorder, and psychotic disorders, as well as sleep medications).

Obviously, not everyone will experience sexual difficulties as a side effect of taking these drugs, and the dysfunction can vary in severity depending on the individual patient, the type of medication, the dosage, the number of medications prescribed for that patient, and their medical condition. Every drug has certain chemical mechanisms of action that can influence any or all aspects of sexual desire and activity. Some drugs will have mixed effects that impact the nervous system differently. There is no simple or "cookbook" approach to this incredibly complex process.

In examining the impact of medications, there are a number of sexual problems that can result. These effects can be the direct result of the chemical mechanisms the drug has on the body, or the sexual side effects can be indirect in nature in that they result from some other drug side effect. The most common sexually related effect of medication is diminished desire, which applies fairly equally to both sexes. The next most frequent direct sexual side effect is erectile difficulties, followed by orgasmic difficulties in both males and females.

The most common orgasmic dysfunction in women is delayed orgasm.[2] Females can also experience lubrication difficulties and menstrual disorders, which can interfere with sexual appetite, function, and frequency. Symptoms of breast enlargement (gynecomastia), lactation, painful sustained erection (priapism), painful intercourse (dyspareunia), infertility, and subnormal testosterone levels (hypogonadism) are less frequent but still quite disturbing when they occur. Certain drugs can even create psychotic delusional states, which can initially manifest as hypersexuality. This is when a person's judgment and perceptions are so distorted they make very poor or dangerous choices.

It is also important to recognize possible indirect sexual side effects that result not from the chemical properties of the drug, but from some other drug effect, such as excessive sleepiness, changes in mood and energy levels, weight loss or gain, or body image. These indirect effects can make a person too sleepy, too unhappy, too tired, or too confused for sex to be appealing or possible. These effects may be the result of neurological factors (e.g., headaches, dizziness, pain, numbness), physical levels of comfort (e.g., constipation, dryness, nausea, indigestion, rash), hormonal in nature (e.g., alterations in insulin metabolism or thyroid function), or a function of vascular problems (e.g., arrhythmias, headaches, vasoconstriction).[3]

There are several popular drugs of abuse that have significant sexual side effects. "Marlboro man" is now "Impotent man" because *smoking* (nicotine) shrinks the blood vessels and decreases blood flow to the brain and to the penis, and causes increased blood flow out of the penis, which results in damage to veins and genital tissue. In addition to causing impotence, it increases arteriosclerosis and impairs testosterone production.[4]

Alcohol stimulates sexual desire at low doses due to disinhibition, but sexual responsiveness is dulled and erection and orgasm are decreased at intoxicating doses. With chronic use, breast enlargement, atrophied testicles, infertility, and feminization may occur in males because testosterone decreases and estrogen increases. It would not be inaccurate to tell male alcoholics that alcohol goes directly to their testicles, causing damage so that their genitals age before they do. In female alcoholics, menstrual disorders, pelvic inflammatory disease, and bleeding disorders are common due to decreased vaginal blood flow and lubrication.[5] Shakespeare was thus cor-

rect those many years ago when he said, "It [drink] pro-
vokes the desire, but it takes away the performance."

The medications used to control high blood pressure
(antihypertensives) have the highest incidence of interfering with erections and ejaculations, as well as having
some impact on sex drive. This is because these drugs
tend to block the norepinephrine activity that is necessary for sexual activation. These drugs are trying to calm
down your overactive system, not add to your excitement. The worst offenders in terms of sexual function are
beta blockers and diuretics. The angiotensin-converting
enzyme (ACE) inhibitors such as captopril (Capoten),
lisinipril (Zestril, Prinivil), and enalapril (Vasotec) appear
to have fewer sexual side effects than many of the other
blood pressure medications.

(*Note:* In listing medications throughout this chapter,
the generic name will be used first and the brand
name(s) will follow in parentheses.)

Antiulcer medications tend to block histamine, which is
excitatory. Cimitadine (Tagamet) is the most sexually
toxic because it interferes with testosterone production.
Ranitadine (Zantac) and famotidine (Pepcid) appear less
likely to have this side effect.

Cold and allergy medications include antihistamines
(e.g., Benadryl) and decongestants (e.g., Sudafed).
Antihistamines can cause sedation and problems with
lubrication. Decongestants can interfere with erections.

Psychiatric medications can also interfere with sexual
function. The antipsychotic drugs block the overactive
dopamine receptors that are creating the psychosis, but
dopamine is necessary for the sexual process to occur.

The newer antipsychotics like olanzapine (Zyprexa), aripiprazole (Abilify), or risperidone (Risperdal) appear to have a lower incidence of sexual dysfunction.[6]

Depression is a very common problem as we get older, especially with the variety of losses that must be managed. As a result, many physicians are often quick to prescribe an antidepressant as a form of treatment. Unfortunately, antidepressants have the highest incidence of inhibiting desire. They can also be associated with orgasmic problems, erectile problems and, occasionally, pain with ejaculation. A very popular class of antidepressant medications is the serotonin selective reuptake inhibitors (SSRIs) like fluoxetine (Prozac), paroxetine (Paxil), sertraline (Zoloft), citalopram (Celexa), and escitalopram (Lexapro). These drugs can cause significant sexual problems because they work to increase serotonin, which helps treat depression but negatively impacts desire, arousal, and orgasm. A potential benefit of the side effect of delayed ejaculation is the use of these medications in the treatment of premature ejaculation. There is a decreased incidence of sexual difficulties associated with the use of nefazadone (Serzone), mirtazapine (Remeron), and fluvoxamine (Luvox). This is especially true for bupropion (Wellbutrin or Zyban) because it stimulates the release of dopamine and norepinephrine and not serotonin.

In general, when possible, it is best to adjust the dosage or change the medication rather than add another one to offset the side effect of the first drug. Inform your physician of any side effects you may be experiencing, so they may be specifically addressed at each visit and adjustments can be made. Non-drug-related methods should be introduced first in order to better minimize expense, additional side effects, and inconvenience. The following are guidelines to consider and discuss with your prescriber in attempting to manage medication-induced sexual dysfunction.[7]

1. *Wait for spontaneous remission of side effects.* Side effects are often more severe in the initial weeks of treatment and later diminish. However, treatment-emergent sexual dysfunction tends to persist.

2. *Decrease the medication to a lower dose.* Sexual dysfunction is often dose-related, so lowering the dose may be helpful, as long as it is not lowered below the therapeutic threshold.

3. *Try partial or complete drug holidays.* This will not work for all medications or in all medical conditions. However, for SSRI-induced sexual dysfunction, reducing or holding the medication for a weekend can reduce or eliminate the dysfunction during that time. This will not work for fluoxetine (Prozac) because it is too long-lasting for this to be effective.

4. *Change to a different medication with fewer sexual side effects.* For example, the antidepressants with the fewest effects on sexual function are bupropion (Wellbutrin), nefazadone (Serzone), venlafaxine (Effexor), and mirtazapine (Remeron). Be cautious in switching from paroxetine (Paxil) or fluoxetine (Prozac) to nefazadone (Serzone) because of a significant drug interaction.

5. *Use a secondary agent to decrease sexual dysfunction.* Adding an adjunctive agent may be possible in many cases, but concern should be given to the possibility of additional side effects or drug interaction concerns. The

following are possible adjunctive agents that may function as sex boosters:

- A low dose of bupropion (Wellbutrin) 75 mg once or twice a day.
- Yohimbine: 5.4–10.8 mg, as needed before intercourse.
- PDE-5 inhibitors (Viagra, Levitra, Cialis): These medications are contraindicated in those with cardiovascular disease or those taking nitrates (such as nitroglycerin).
- Cyproheptadine (Periactin): 4–12 mg one to two hours prior to intercourse.
- Dopamine-stimulating drugs and psychostimulants: Amantadine (Symmetrel) 100–200 mg once a day; Lisuride, bromocriptine (Parlodel), dextroamphetamine (Dexedrine), and methylphenidate (Ritalin) have all been used with varying success.
- Ginkgo biloba: 60–180 mg twice a day may be effective in sexual dysfunction due to limited blood flow in the genitals. Side effects include gastrointestinal disturbances, headache, and general central nervous system activation.[8]

SEXUAL BOOSTERS

I recently saw a bumper sticker that said, "I'm on Prozac, Rogaine, and Viagra—I'm happy, hairy, and horny." We live in an era where we are seeing major developments in the treatment of sexual dysfunction. However, when it comes to the "sex boosters," the PDE-5 inhibitors, or impotence pills, are stealing the headlines (as well as the advertising dollars). The three medications currently being marketed are sildenafil (Viagra), vardenafil (Levitra), and tadalafil (Cialis). These pills are taken orally before lovemaking and help the penis respond to stimulation. The medication enhances the action of cyclic GMP (a chemical released in the production of nitric oxide in the nerve cells surrounding the penis, which has the effect of widening the blood vessels in the penis). Cyclic GMP inhibits the effect of phosphoresterase 5 or PDE 5, an enzyme that is abundant in impotent men that blocks arousal.[9] Interestingly, there is increasing evidence that these medications may help improve blood flow and lubrication in the vaginal and clitoral area for women.

These drugs only work in the context of desire and physical stimulation, so it won't work if you slip it into your husband's coffee. They are truly "spirit is willing, but the flesh is weak" drugs. An improved ability to perform, however, can create confidence and greater desire. This class of drugs all work similarly in the body, although there may be some difference as to the length of time each pill works actively. Viagra tends to be effective for about two to three hours, Levitra for about five hours, and Cialis for up to twenty-four to thirty-six hours. The marketing claims that Levitra and Cialis can work within twenty to thirty minutes and Viagra after about an hour, but some men will respond in less than one hour. Men taking nitrate drugs (often used to control chest pain, also known as angina) should not take these medications because of the possibility of a rapid and dangerous drop in blood pressure. The most common side effects include headache, flushing, and stuffy or runny nose.

Be cautious about the dangers of ordering PDE-5 inhibitors over the Internet if you have not had a medical evaluation from your physician or do not have a current prescription. Men who are physically unfit, have underlying cardiac problems, have liver or kidney impairment, or suffer from severe arterial insufficiency (blood flow problems) may find the medication does not work for them or may create a medical emergency. The possibility of a prolonged painful erection (priapism) can lead to the risk of permanent impotence.

An additional note and caution should be considered regarding the abundance of over-the-counter, herbal, and other Internet products touted as "all-natural alternatives." These substances are typically not regulated by the FDA, and rarely are there replicated studies on their effectiveness and safety. These products are often combined with various other ingredients, such as Yohimbine, L-arginine, DHEA, Ginkgo biloba, and Korean ginseng. But are the combination products safe? They may be for many, but they are not safe for people with hypertension, other heart conditions or anxiety, or for people on the blood thinner Warfarin.

Remember, all medications, herbal supplements, and vitamins have side effects. Be an informed consumer. Wisely get medical advice from more than one source, and research the Internet or library. Work together with your partner as you seek to maximize the benefit of medications and minimize their sexual side effects. Understanding the impact of medications will allow you (and your doctor) to make the adjustments necessary to enhance your relational intimacy.

Chapter 11

The Viagra Years:
Blessing or Curse?

*V*iagra has been termed by Erica Jong "the perfect American medication" because "it raises the Dow Jones and the penis too." The impotence pills and the enormous publicity surrounding them tell us a lot about the values in our culture. Sales of Viagra were roughly $437 million in the third quarter of 2002. Analysts estimate the impotence market will increase from the $1.6 billion today to between $3 billion and $4 billion a year by 2006.[1] The advent of Viagra has undoubtedly had a major impact on the thirty million men in the United States (and 150 million men worldwide) with erectile dysfunction. It has been received with pleasure by many older couples as a partner has been able to experience revitalized sexual function. These

PDE-5 inhibitors have become a standard treatment intervention to aid in the erectile recovery for men who have nerve-sparing prostatectomies. These medications can also be helpful for men with psychological impotence, as they can boost confidence and aid in breaking the performance-anxiety cycle.

However, utilizing medical manipulation to enhance the performance of a man's penis will not heal a relationship that is not working. I remember one person telling me [Jim], "I can get it up now, but I still don't want to have sex with her." The focus of this chapter will be to examine the impact of Viagra and similar drugs (Levitra and Cialis) on relationships. In Chapter 5 we referred to the problems inherent in the "sexual performance perfection industry" of which Viagra may be symbolic. It is a commentary on our society that focuses on the penis and genitals and the importance of enhanced performance and functioning versus the process of developing mature intimacy.

POSSIBLE CONSEQUENCES FOR RELATIONSHIPS

The rapid return of sexual function in one partner will create problems if the other partner does not want to resume sexual relations. This can be true of a woman who may be secretly relieved her husband is impotent because she had adjusted to a life without sex, and avoiding sex was a fine way to avoid intimacy. Some couples who had become comfortable as "affectionate roommates" and had learned to cope with and accept the impotency, now may have to learn how to respond to his renewed potency.

This may require an open and honest dialogue between the couple as to how to change the status quo.

Some women may be willing to become sexually active again but find their bodies uncooperative. A woman who has been postmenopausal for several years will not find it easy to suddenly resume intercourse. Thinning vaginal walls and diminished lubrication will require a cooperative and patient response from the husband. She will need to slowly ease back into sex, and her husband will need to appreciate and understand this adjustment. He needs to remember that even though he now has the capacity for an erect penis, he will need to take the time to court his bride and practice seducing her again. This is not the time for increased expectations and demands.[2]

Viagra-like drugs can also create a crisis for a man if his wife expects him to be able to return to sexual functioning, and he no longer has an "excuse" to avoid being sexually intimate with her. The advent of these drugs may thus precipitate an uncovering of relational problems long swept under the rug. Remember, these medications restore the capacity for an erection but do not increase libido. They are not aphrodisiacs and require a partner's active participation. A man who is depressed, angry, stressed, or hurt will not find a magical solution to his problems by popping this pill.

Some men will take their newly discovered erections and be prone to wander in an attempt to find a more willing companion. There may be a flurry of affairs and divorces that result from differing expectations and unmet needs. Some of the same groups vulnerable to affairs in general are made more so by Viagra: (1) *Men having midlife crises:* A man insecure in his sexuality may look for the fast car, younger woman, and the erection he had when he was eighteen. (2) *Couples facing the empty nest:* The kids have left home and the couple are faced for the first time in years with being "just with each other." (3) *Wives going through menopause:* She's adjusting to physical and emotional changes and may have a decreased interest in sex.[3] It is also not unusual to find older men with unwilling partners having relationships with available middle-aged women. Again, the impotence pills may force some couples to face relational problems they have long been ignoring. This may be quite troubling and result in more distance for some couples. But for others, these drugs may help them strengthen their marriage by pushing them to resolve issues in their marriage.

The impotence pills remind us again that a healthy marriage and intimate lovemaking are about connection and not penetration. It's not about the penis, but about the person and the ability to connect intimately.

CONNECTING VERSUS PENETRATING

As you lie with your mate and experience the intimacy of holding hands, caressing faces, hugging close, and stimulating sexual excitement, you are energized and affirmed. Making love provides a safe haven that you can delight in despite the environmental pressures. As you age, this becomes even more important, and your sex life is symbolic of your ability to still be in charge of your marriage and your destiny. But the vast majority of older males continue to believe that all sexual expression must involve penile-vaginal penetration. The Viagra-like drugs have the tendency to change a man's ego and reinforce the performance orientation of our society. Many of these same men may believe that the interpersonal relationship should have little influence on their ability to have an erection. These beliefs are recipes for sexual and relational disaster.

As we age, we can mature in our concepts of lovemaking. If sex is to be a celebration, we need to have a relationship to celebrate, and this is more true than ever as we grow older. If a couple develops their abilities to connect and communicate, and acquires many ways to achieve intimacy besides just sexual intercourse, they have a healthy repertoire to draw on when disease or disability strikes. They have a much greater ability to successfully adapt to changes inherent in the aging process, because they have developed their understanding of making love.

NURTURING EACH OTHER'S SPIRIT

M. Scott Peck, in his best-selling book *The Road Less Traveled,* defines *love* as "the will to extend oneself for the purpose of nurturing one's own or another's spiritual growth."[4] This definition challenges us to put love into action and begs us to answer two questions if we are to be good "lovers." First, what is it that nurtures my own or my spouse's growth? Not just what arouses them or makes them temporarily feel good, but how can my nurturance make a difference in his or her life? The second question to consider is: What areas in my life or my spouse's life are in need of additional growth? The ability to communicate? The ability to resolve conflict? Unresolved issues with family or friends? Relationship with God? There may be many areas of potential growth, and each of them will *enhance* my ability to legitimately love my spouse.

My ability to better nurture my spouse will manifest itself in the bedroom as we celebrate the effort we have put into our relationship. In aging, bodies do not respond with the same reflexive arousal but need the attention and nurturing of a partner in special ways. Older mates feel a greater sense of mutuality and power in their love-making. A husband may need his wife to stimulate his penis into an erection and help him reach a climax in ways he did not in earlier years. This can be very exciting and bonding to a wife as she enjoys being more aggressive and playful in her sexuality. Her husband involves and counts on her more, and she enjoys this form of nurturing. A man may acquire greater tenderness, sensitivity, and patience that make him a much more adept lover. Couples have fun feeling needed and engaging in mutual nurturing with a deeper sense of connection. They appreciate being skilled and generous lovers.

God desires us to mature and gain wisdom with age. Sex can become even more special after age fifty and sixty and even eighty. Mature men and women are even better equipped, mentally and emotionally and physically, to bring their intimate companion and themselves greater pleasure. Your fulfilling partnership can achieve a level never before experienced, and your lovemaking can be an integral part of that whole process. In this context, Viagra-like drugs may well be a blessing. However, without a mutual participation in this "dance of intimacy," they very well may function as a curse.

Chapter 12

Challenges and Choices:
Sexual Desire and Frequency

I am so frustrated; sex used to be the exciting glue in our companionship, and now I hardly ever think about it." Problems of sexual desire[1] are the most common presenting concern that brings couples into sex therapy (and marital therapy for sexual issues). A survey of more than two thousand Christian women, the National Study on the Sexuality of Christian Women (NSSCW), found one in three married women experiencing difficulty feeling sexual desire.[2] Menopause, illnesses, medications, and adjusting to changing bodies and roles all create many challenges in the mature years.

Some problems have simple answers: Sell the boat, move nearer the grandkids, learn golf. *In desire issues, there are usually multiple, multilayered causes with both partners contributing uniquely to the problem.* A complexity of issues along many fronts must be addressed. Creative solutions do exist, but let's unpack some of the complexity of the issue as we define *desire* and explore some broad categories of challenges around inhibited desire—with possible solutions.

DEFINING *DESIRE*

Couples that come for help with desire issues provide a wide range of standards and expectations of normal sexual desire and frequency. Many men set their own sexual desire as the standard their wife must meet. Others pull from friends, media, or culture. Failure to meet the standard they have adopted is interpreted as an inadequacy in themselves or their spouse. Unfortunately, the standards people choose are rarely appropriate standards.

The way the media have depicted sex has added a great deal of pressure and false expectations. The truth is that sexual desire is three-dimensional and stems from our bodies (hormones, genitals, seeing, and touching), our souls (emotions, minds, fantasy, choices), and our spirits (attraction and commitment). In media sex, partners easily become aroused, and everyone has fantastic orgasms. With these expectations ingrained in each of us, a genuine sexual relationship in the real world will most likely produce feelings of inferiority and dissatisfaction. One or both partners begin to wonder, *What is wrong with us?* The normal aspects of aging can quickly trigger these feelings.

Gender Differences

Husbands and wives will rarely (if ever) have the same sexual desire. Most experts and studies state that men have a more apparent and assertive desire, but it is a myth that men are always hormonally driven and can instantly get erections. Men, too, get tired, have difficulty being aroused, and can struggle with getting erections for a variety of reasons and lose their sexual desire.

However, the complexity of sexual desire in women cannot be underestimated. Many elements can sabotage a woman's sexual desire: her physical health, energy level, whether or not she is depressed, hormones, how she feels about her appearance, how she perceives her marriage partner, how distracted she is by other concerns, whether or not she has been sexually abused, how her family of origin viewed sexuality, any medications she is taking, and whether or not sex has been or has become painful—physically or emotionally. All of these factors and their interactions combine to create, enhance, or diminish a woman's sexual desire.

Types of Desire

Sexual desire can be thought of as having three varieties: assertive, receptive, or low. Assertive desire is more typical of men with a longing to seek out sex. This type of desire more actively thinks about sexual activity and initiates sexual connection with a physical drive. A more feminine flavor of assertive desire occurs with what can be termed "alluring" desire. This is typical of the wife who enjoys the feminine power of her body and nature for enticing and turning her husband on sexually.

Receptive desire is more typical of women and includes an openness to sexual activity, enjoying the closeness, and getting involved, often after initiation. Sexual thoughts and arousal may come to the wife after she begins to engage in lovemaking, with an internal response of *I wasn't thinking of sex tonight but, wow, this was a good idea.* A flavor of receptive desire emerges as "nurturing" desire. This desire comes to the forefront when a mate may not want lovemaking for him or herself, but wants to give fulfillment as a gift to the partner.

Normal Desire

It is important to realize that "low" sexual desire can be a relative and arbitrary term. Most couples experience desire discrepancy, but both may be normal with one partner having a "high" normal desire and the other a "low" normal desire. Remember the statistical bell-shaped curve:

Fig. 12.1

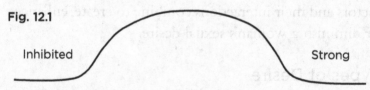

Inhibited   Strong

You probably have heard some story of a woman who wanted sex all the time. We call this the "nympho myth," and yet 68 percent of women will fall along the middle or average part of the desire curve (see Figure 12.1). Another 14 percent will have either lower or higher desire, with only 2 percent being on the extremes. Wives are often quite average in desire, and the husband doesn't have to be a sexual machine.

HOW DESIRE IS CHALLENGED AND ENHANCED

Here are five broad categories that trigger low sexual desire. Each of these categories could be a whole book. Be a detective and apply these general problem areas to your specific desire issues.

1. Body Busters and Boosters

The human body is wonderfully complex. It is important to remember that most illnesses as well as the normal process of aging affect the body and can take a real toll on sexual desire. All medications and drugs have side effects and many have some sexual side effects. In several chapters throughout this book, we have considered the effects of aging on hormones. Read these chapters and practice some of the creative solutions we suggest.

2. Emotional Toxins and Antidotes

Our positive emotions are vital to sexual arousal. Other types of feelings can be quite toxic to desire, as they have serious negative impact on our personal and relational well-being. Certain emotions must be resolved and worked through for sexual desire to return. A central theme of this book is working through the many normal feelings that will be evoked in the aging process.

Depression, Loss, and Grief. Depression, with its accompanying loss of energy and mood changes and irritability, affects sexual desire and frequency. As negative as the depression itself is, antidepressants often have an inhibitory impact on arousal or orgasm, which can further complicate desire. Grief has a tremendous impact on intimacy in general and lovemaking in particular. One husband in counseling wondered what had happened to his sex drive. In exploring recent losses, he had lost a dad to cancer and retired from his job. Any serious loss can certainly contribute to depression and loss of energy and libido.

Fear. In a culture that adores youth and success and ignores those who struggle, fear can be very restricting to sexual desire—and difficult to accept, explore, and understand. The fear of appearing inadequate or incompetent, or the fear of the effects of aging on the body, can quickly dampen sexual initiative. People can be particularly sensitive to sexual pressure and fear. The fear of failure in a partner's eyes is enough to hinder anyone's desire to even try to be sexual.

Anger, Resentment, Disappointment, and Hurt. How can you not step on one of these land mines of feelings as you continually work through the process of aging? It may be a disfiguring surgery, loss of erections, saying good-bye to a tight tummy, or lacking stamina that triggers one of these emotions.

The **antidote** is to dispute the toxic feelings with a healing emotional connection. The following suggestions can do wonders in overcoming the negative emotions mentioned above.

- *Express tender emotions.* Cuddling, massage, and verbally emphasizing caring feelings for each other can be redemptive in countering depression, fear, anger, and hurt.

- *Tell yourself the truth.* In their excellent book *Telling Yourself the Truth,* Backus and Chapian talk about being able to mentally dispute feelings and work through to a positive place.[3] Aging evokes feelings, but we can choose not to allow them to rule our lives as we work through them to a place of acceptance and control.
- *Laugh!* "A cheerful heart is good medicine" (Prov. 17:22 NIV). Laughter has a way of giving perspective, secreting natural painkillers in the brain, and helps to create a connection between partners. It's a great antidote to our discouraging emotions, and the great thing is that maturity gives us a greater ability to laugh at ourselves and life.

3. Personal Brakes and Accelerators

How partners initiate sexual activity, sights, sounds, smells, words that are said (or not said), location, time of day, pace, and a host of other factors can be listed as personal brakes or accelerators of sexual desire. As was developed in the beginning of the chapter, desire is three-dimensional and involves our bodies, our emotions and minds, and our spirits. Each of these three dimensions can be important in understanding the complexity of the brakes and accelerators. Here are some examples of the common brakes with possible accelerators in sex after age fifty.

Fatigue and Timing. One of the surprising discoveries in the NSSCW (Hart et al., 1998) was that lack of sexual desire was not the most frequently cited sexual difficulty. Forty-five percent of the married women said their greatest difficulty was finding the energy for sex. If you're not a night person or are stiff in the morning, aging will exacerbate these characteristics. Make choices and set priorities to overcome fatigue and practice good timing.

Attractiveness and Body Image. Two-thirds of the married women in the NSSCW specifically identified their body image and weight concerns as impacting their sexual desire.[4] Women are masters of comparison, which leads to insecurity, body loathing, anxiety, depression, and a belief they are not attractive to their husbands.

Men also can struggle with their body image with its sags and lost muscle tone. Probably an even greater personal brake that must be worked through is the dramatic changes they see taking place in their wife's body. A husband is more visual but can learn to enjoy a new type of sensuality and erotic arousal. Nipples, labia, and vaginas are very arousing in sixty-, seventy-, or eighty-year-old bodies—especially as sensuality expands beyond body parts to tender touches, erotic caressing, and emotional closeness.

Traumatic Sexual Experiences and Inhibitions. *Sexual trauma* is anything that disrupts healthy sexual development, bringing distortion and inhibition to personal sexuality and married lovemaking. Perimenopause and menopause may cause unresolved issues (family background, abuse, religious prohibitions, fear of relaxing control) to resurface that need to be reworked through to resolution. Get some counseling and face some of those secrets.

In overcoming the personal brakes on desire, many of the **accelerators** are commonsense interventions: take a nap before lovemaking, practice putting the soul into sex as bodies are enjoyed in new ways, learn to communicate, and get some outside help.

4. Relationship Bombs and Builders

A couple's companionship can be a microcosm of what happens in their sex life, and vice versa (see Chapter 7). Marital conflict, boredom, and disrespect often intensify the lack of desire. Traditional marital therapy techniques of teaching forgiveness, assertiveness, communication skills, and conflict resolution skills, as well as working through control issues, can be important when addressing the problems that dump on sexual desire.

Growing old together is not always easy. Midlife crises and their many changes don't always bring with them the resolve to take the high road. Here are some challenges that must be resolved for sexual desire and "feeling in love" to return.

Conflict and Distance. Shrill, angry wives and passively angry husbands with continued power struggles or unresolved issues have a very negative impact on sexuality. Lovemaking reflects whether a couple like each other, are intimate companions, or have many unresolved conflicts.

Extramarital Affairs and Other Distractions. Affairs and other ways of adulterating marital companionship can be common in midlife crises, retirement, and the empty-nest years. Society trivializes adultery, but there is no more powerful way to sabotage sexual wholeness and the hope for true intimacy. Put in place needed boundaries and get therapy to resolve hurts and distancing.

Inertia. An object at rest tends to stay at rest and dig a deeper rut, while one in motion will stay in motion. This law certainly applies to a sex life too. If a couple make love once a month, it is easy to slip into once every three months. Don't buy into the myth that couples in their fifties and older don't make love with frequency. Find those optimal times weekly and stay lovers.

Polarization. As couples wrestle with sexual desire difficulties, often they begin to polarize: One partner feels they have sex "hardly ever," and the other believes they have sex "all the time." One mate will feel emotionally neglected, and the other will feel sexually deprived. Conflict can escalate with mates living in each other's debit column and focusing on shortcomings. A negative pattern develops that further inhibits sexual desire.

Here are three relationship **builders** that can help you rev up a sex life where you may not have made love in months or years:

1. *Start with rebuilding the companionship.* Do some playful, nonsexual activities together.

2. *Increase your nonsexual touch and physical affection.* Oxytocin is a peptide secreted in the brain that flows to various parts of the brain and throughout the reproductive organs of both men and women. It rises in response to touch and promotes touching. Oxytocin effects are increased by estrogen, which has led researchers to hypothesize that oxytocin may be especially important in sexual desire in women. Without touch, oxytocin production falls, as does the bonding in the relationship, lowering sexual desire even further.[5]

3. Make love more frequently. It may take some effort and a few failed attempts to get back to a more consistent sex life. Start with sensual massage, tune in to sexual sensations, and then include a lot of love play and nude hugs and showers before attempting intercourse. As with jumping into cold lake water on a warm, summer day, you eventually must hold your breath, psych yourselves up, and jump into having intercourse. Go into it with no expectation other than breaking the ice. Orgasms aren't necessary. Set a date night to relax and *choose* to make love.

5. Environmental Hazards and Healers

Sexual desire can also be blocked and dumped on by our religious and family values, societal myths, and factors out of our control. These must be understood, disputed, and healed. Here are some common environmental hazards.

Expectations and Myths. Myths abound about sex in the mature years. We have sought to dispel many of these misbeliefs throughout this book. One couple confessed in counseling that they both believed that love-making would totally stop at age sixty. Sure enough, from their midfifties on it slowed down and was gone by sixty. Expectations of more time spent in romance, balanced time around the children's needs, or increased sexual variety must be talked through, or resentment can build and desire will be affected.

Parental Models. Your parents teach you about sex and relationships. They model the ability to be affectionate and affirming. Families openly and subtly impart values to you about sex and trust and self-esteem. Your relationship with your family and parents, even if they are deceased, has an ongoing impact on your current sexual relationship. Discuss this with your siblings or a counselor as you grow and heal some of these attitudes.

Religious and Societal Prohibitions. Sex is a gift from God, but you couldn't prove it by many people raised in Christian homes and the church. Sex was never talked about and was treated with such hesitation and avoidance that they are afraid of sexual intimacy.

Powerful **healing** influences can be appropriated when the environment has dumped on and squelched sexual desire.

Undertake Renewing Your Mind. Identify the erroneous messages about sex in your head and challenge them with truth. Do a lot of self-talk. You might say, "Relax . . . it's okay . . . enjoy . . . play at it." Create positive affirmation statements: "God created sexual pleasure"; "I am capable of change"; "If I enjoy sex, it does not mean I will lose control"; "Sex is fun, and I don't need to feel guilty anymore."

Pray! Sexuality and sexual expression were God's idea and His gift to us. When we, or those we try to help, encounter sexual problems, we need to turn to God for help, hope, and healing. We can practice praying, individually and together, for the growth and health of our sexual relationship.

Low sexual desire is truly a complex puzzle, but *sexual intimacy is not just an option if you want to remain lovers.* Be courageous and assertive in not settling for low desire and unsatisfying, infrequent lovemaking. Find those creative solutions.

Chapter 13

"Why Didn't I Say That?"
Choosing to Communicate Sexually

$\mathcal{O}$ne would hope that with maturity would come an easier ability to dialogue about sex. Unfortunately, creating a comfortable sexual vocabulary and developing the skills to communicate about lovemaking don't come easy at any age. Remember the formula and the need to face the challenges of these mature years and choose to create a great love life.

Creative Solutions

↗

Changes → Challenges → Choices

↘

Negative Existence

In order to celebrate lovemaking after age fifty, we must take greater initiative to communicate about and work toward creative solutions, or we may end up settling for an intimacy-deprived partnership. For example, Stan needs more direct stimulation to become aroused. Sally enjoys more gentle intercourse with simultaneous massage of her back. The following keys of empathy and coaching will help you become mature communicators.

EMPATHY: THE KEY TO GREAT COMMUNICATION

The essence of effective communication is a dialogue that ends in empathy. One partner has assertively stated his or her reality, and the other partner has been able to walk in his or her shoes to understand and acknowledge that reality. Empathy is all about understanding. It is *not agreeing*, but rather hearing and acknowledging another reality that often differs from our own.

A crucial part of effective communication and avoiding defensiveness is coming into this process with a deeply loving attitude that conveys to the mate, "I like you—you're safe with me; I want you happy and fulfilled." Mature communicators in this dialogue process abandon the need to *win, debate, convince,* or *make a point.* You are creating a dialogue with the goal of exchanging data. Each partner communicates his or her reality while the other listens and works through to empathy.

1. Assertively *State* Your Personal Reality

Start with "I" statements that take responsibility without blaming (not "You turn me off," but "I feel my desire shut down when you grab at me"). Assertive communication is direct and respectful without being aggressive or passive. Risk conflict and express your core feelings and needs. Don't get hung up on one point but express the greater reality and what's going on gut-level. You are communicating information that your mate really needs in order to have a contented spouse. Share that data!

Practice Exercise: In a self-aware, honest manner, communicate to your mate how you have changed sexually as you have aged and what you desire more of in your present lovemaking. Complete the following sentence: "I wish sexually that you would . . ." or "I enjoy it when you . . ." Then dialogue about your answers.

2. Objectively *Empathize* with Your Partner's Reality

Express understanding of your partner's message with short empathy summaries. Go beyond the surface content to acknowledge the deeper needs and feelings. Remember that empathy is not agreeing that your mate's reality is free of distortions or accepting their feelings as correct and true. It is containing your judgments and feelings while you try to understand his or her reality. You may speak German and have to learn some French to really empathize correctly. Be aware that your mate *will not feel heard* until he or she has felt empathy and understanding. (*A note for husbands:* Wives especially need to have the feeling part of their reality empathized with and acknowledged. They can be like a broken record that keeps repeating itself until you have empathized with their feelings.)

Practice Exercise: Ask your partner to describe a love-making session that was very special. Put yourself in your mate's sexual reality, and decide what some of his or her deeper needs are (e.g., variety, tenderness, competence, challenge, affirmation, fun, comfort). Use remarks like: "What I'm hearing is . . ." or "You must feel . . ." or "You're needing me to . . ." Switch roles and let your partner convey his or her reality.

3. Tenderly *Negotiate* a Partnership Reality

Create tentative solutions. Bargain with the collected data of each reality, as both lovingly compromise. The purpose of dialogue is to mutually meet needs and resolve differences, not to win or make your point. This may mean to agree to disagree while you work on thinking through an issue more, while temporarily putting it on hold. It could mean a behavioral solution negotiated around each mate's needs and feelings, a solution both are willing to try to implement even though it may end up being 20-80 or 40-60. Few compromises are 50-50, but with dialogue and empathy with each other's souls—it still feels like a compromise even if only 20 percent of your needs are met this time.

In your solutions, neither of you must lose your soul as you lovingly compromise. What I mean by losing your souls is that if a mate compromises on certain issues, they will lose an important part of who they are and their deeper values. Love is patient, kind, and protective. Paraphrasing Matthew 16:26, what does it profit a mate if they gain their own way but their partner loses his or her soul? For example, a husband realized his wife would run the risk of another yeast infection if she gave in to his desire to give her oral sex, so he wisely gave up this request.

Practice Exercise: Each of you take the data you have collected and propose a tentative solution around a challenge in your sex life. Make sure neither of you loses his or her soul but also realize that what goes around comes around in good relationships. The 20-80 compromises even out over time in loving, giving partnerships.

THE LANGUAGE OF LOVEMAKING

Each partnership will benefit from erotic communication. A fun part of your fifties and beyond can be feeling comfortable enough with yourselves and each other to finally develop your sexual vocabulary—both verbal and nonverbal.

Vocabulary and Slang

In developing a sexual vocabulary, you may be wondering if slang is ever appropriate. Of course; slang is permissible and fun and erotic. Your pet names for body parts and secret vocabulary shared by only the two of you contain a lot of slang. And as a couple you will find other words expressive and arousing. As Christians, however, we must be careful to avoid the very negative attitudes and ideas about sex that society over the centuries has incorporated into slang. *We never want to be funny at someone's expense, harmfully aggressive, demeaning to our partners, or cheaply suggestive.*

You should know the correct biological terms for

parts of the human body. That is a good starting point. Learn to converse openly about making love without shame or embarrassment, and talk during sex. Expand your vocabulary, and adapt slang that both of you enjoy. Sex is your playground, and great communication translates into having more fun.

Time Out: Have fun the next time you are making love by creating some pet names for activities and body parts. (I often laugh in counseling sessions when clients talk about "Big John" or "Shamu" and wanting to "dive into your pool, but you fell asleep.") Tell your mate of two slang words you find exciting and two that you feel would decrease your sexual enjoyment and arousal.

Nonverbal Signals

Build an arousing and useful repertoire of nonverbal language. Experts speculate that anywhere from 65 to 95 percent of communication is nonverbal, so it is no wonder that great lovers master this aspect of connecting. Perhaps gentle pressure with a hand signals the desire to shift into another position. Groans, sighs, and exclamations may signal degrees of arousal and when to proceed to another phase of lovemaking. Nonverbal communication helps orchestrate a sex life that will grow ever more comfortable and meaningful.

Develop nonverbal signals that indicate your desire for

sexual activity. Without allowing it to completely lose its subtlety, make sure the nonverbal vocabulary is accurate and obvious enough. It may be a passionate hug or kiss. Sometimes an amorous look or a soft kiss on the back of the neck is all it takes. A husband related that his wife usually initiated her desire for sex with a certain nightgown. He thought the nonverbal signal was okay, but he wished after eight years she would buy another gown.

Nonverbal communication evolves with most lovers, and growing older is a great time to trust yourself to be uninhibited and playful. Don't just use nonverbal signals to direct lovemaking, but give yourself permission to be uninhibited and make noises during sex. Groan, breathe loudly, exclaim in excitement, purr with pleasure, squeal with delight, and allow your nonverbal communication to be truly expressive.

Coaching

Coaching involves assertively expressing your sexual needs and feelings, learning to problem-solve around difficult areas, and *helping your mate understand you.* You can't immediately know exactly all the things that pleasure or turn off your partner. These change with the aging process and demand constant readjustment with effective coaching.

Here are some important guidelines for giving helpful suggestions as you coach your mate and find creative solutions for enhancing your sex life:

1. *Major coaching should be done away from the bedroom.* Dialogue about your sex life could include the subjects of poor hygiene, physical changes, inhibitions around

body image, boredom, pushiness, and/or technique deficits. For example, "I would really appreciate you brushing your teeth more regularly." "I feel more comfortable having my scars covered during lovemaking."

2. Minor coaching adjustments utilize nonverbal and verbal language that can be done nonthreateningly during lovemaking. For example, "That hurts." "Slow down." "You're on my arm." "More." "Shift."

3. Focus on the positive! The primary goal of coaching is not simply to correct what's wrong—it is to maximize the strengths and bring out the best.

Initiating and Refusing

All successful lovers polish initiating and refusing. People and their needs change with a proneness for misunderstandings in this area of sexual communication.

- "I wish we could make love at a time of day when I feel fresher."
- "I'm not always ready to make love as my wife expects."

Even in later stages of life and long-term relationships, initiating and refusing remain symbolic and filled with disappointments and hurt feelings. First, initiating and refusing make one vulnerable to rejection and feelings of abandonment. Second, much of initiating is nonverbal and therefore open to misinterpretation. Third, initiating, or the lack thereof, becomes synonymous with sexual desire and sexual attractiveness. Fourth, initiating sex means coordinating two unique people with different needs.

Time Out: Switch roles. Role-play being your mate and demonstrate how you would like him or her to initiate and refuse lovemaking with you. In this positive way you remember your mate's reality, as you coach your mate on the things you appreciate and the things you would like to see eliminated. Practice both nonverbal and verbal techniques as you smooth the process and make it honest and loving.

We cannot stress enough the importance of communication skills in working through the constant challenges and choices of the mature years. Read a book, watch a video, listen to an audiotape, or take a class together on improving communication in your marriage. Your love life will be the winner with more effective communication and coaching.

Chapter 14

From Here to Eternity: *Understanding the Lovemaking Cycle*

*I*n the silver and golden years of marriage, lovemaking can grow ever more meaningful. What an amazing connection occurs as you look deeply into the eyes and soul of your lover, and playfully, vulnerably stir up in each other the passion, sensuality, and mystery of sexuality. God has designed a marvelously complex and intimate cycle to be set in motion when a couple make love. This chapter will describe a model that considers the increasing emotional and relational intimacy that builds during lovemaking.

THE LOVEMAKING CYCLE

Christian sex therapist Christopher McCluskey has created a relational and emotional Lovemaking Cycle.[1] He insists that there is a great deal of difference between "having sex" and "making love." True lovemaking (the cycle) creates a growing intimacy and an increasing sexual passion based on two hearts becoming spiritually and emotionally one.

In McCluskey's model, each part of the cycle feeds into the next, creating an ever-deepening experience of vulnerability and intimacy with your mate and lover. He emphasizes that if one part is neglected, lovemaking will "clunk" every time it hits that weak spot and will throw off the whole cycle—much like a wheel that is flat in one area and no longer round. Lovemaking will in time break down because each of the four parts represents a deep emotional and relational need that is critical for maintaining passionate lovemaking.

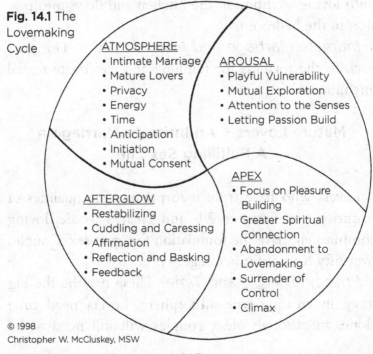

Fig. 14.1 The Lovemaking Cycle

ATMOSPHERE
• Intimate Marriage
• Mature Lovers
• Privacy
• Energy
• Time
• Anticipation
• Initiation
• Mutual Consent

AROUSAL
• Playful Vulnerability
• Mutual Exploration
• Attention to the Senses
• Letting Passion Build

AFTERGLOW
• Restabilizing
• Cuddling and Caressing
• Affirmation
• Reflection and Basking
• Feedback

APEX
• Focus on Pleasure Building
• Greater Spiritual Connection
• Abandonment to Lovemaking
• Surrender of Control
• Climax

© 1998
Christopher W. McCluskey, MSW

This model identifies many important factors that can facilitate progressively deeper levels of intimacy in love-making. Each will be briefly examined and explained, with an emphasis on the four key areas that are truly interactive and must flow through the heart: atmosphere, arousal, apex, and afterglow.

Stage 1: Atmosphere

Mood setting can never be simply lighting a candle or creating a little ambience. *The concept of atmosphere is much deeper.* It is lovingly building an intimate relationship with your covenant companion so that energy is reserved and time is devoted for sexuality. Time, energy, and anticipation are powerful aphrodisiacs. Desire is never just hormonal, especially for the wife. Sex begins with loving attention in the kitchen and flows into passion in the bedroom.

Intimate Marriage and Mature Lovers. This goes back to the formula for fulfilling and passionate sexual encounters:

**Mature Lovers + An Intimate Marriage =
A Fulfilling Sex Life**

Lovers who have truly incorporated the qualities of maturity (see Chapter 20) and created a safe, loving commitment have the foundation for great sex. Couples over fifty have a distinct edge.

Privacy, Energy, and Time. These may be the big three in creating true atmosphere. Lovers need time alone, and though older couples will still need to be aware of distractions, more opportunities for intimate time exist with the empty nest and a greater focus on quality of life. Time may be the most precious gift you bring to your sex life. It is the bottom line in creating the sensual, connected atmosphere as you get beyond quickies to luxuriating. Five-second hugs, lingering, deep kisses, and two-hour picnics in bed will do wonders. Reserving some energy for sex may be a greater challenge, but taking an extra nap or allowing some recreational time can be creatively arranged if it's a priority. Rest and recreation create energy.

Anticipation. Great lovers are childlike in their ability to anticipate pleasure with glee. Husbands and especially wives can enjoy their God-given imagination and think about lovemaking more—like a kid who has looked forward to an ice-cream cone all day.

Initiation and Mutual Consent. Lovemaking has to start somewhere, and a part of atmosphere is both husband and wife mutually initiating sexual activity. Remember, it does not have to lead to intercourse but can be that gentle kiss or tender caress. Older lovers often let romance and sexuality permeate the relationship in an easy, comfortable manner. Their lovemaking may consist of that knowing glance or light touch as initiation and mutual movement toward each other create atmosphere.

Stage 2: Arousal

Sexual maturity helps us grow beyond the arousal of sexual rushes and buzzes. Deep, erotic arousal grows from a three-dimensional connection and bonding of body, soul, and spirit. When you and your mate learn to be aroused in this truly *intimate* way, you will be amazed at the feelings that occur. The physical and emotional interaction and fusion (God-given eros) create an unbeatable intimacy high.

Playful Vulnerability. Fun and open lovemaking takes place in the child-ego state. Each of us has that curious, silly, innocent, playful part of us that loves to romp. God gave imaginations and the ability to be romantic to create and enjoy various means of enticing and playing with our mates. Maturity can make us more creative. "Naked and unashamed" is a very vulnerable and powerful place to be (cf. Chapter 1 and playfulness).

Mutual Exploration. Learn the hot spots and the turnoffs. As we age these may change. What delightful lovemaking occurs when you can help your mate discover an arousing spot they weren't aware of or experience a new situation that helps them to be comfortable and gets them excited. An attitude of exploration keeps lovemaking fresh.

Attention to the Senses. Every individual and couple could profit by tuning in to how each of their senses cues them in to sexual arousal—how they want that sense to be utilized. Observe and make a list of what turns you on with each sense and what detracts from lovemaking. Some of these sensual items may already be in your normal lovemaking routines; some you may wish to creatively add or delete (turnoffs). A sample list might include:

Sight	Turn-ons: Soft bed, nighties, silk boxers, nakedness

	Turnoffs: Bright lights, being ungroomed, dirty sheets
Smell	Turn-ons: Candles, scented lotions, semen, cologne
	Turnoffs: Body odor, dirty sheets, semen
Taste	Turn-ons: Minty kisses, a favorite wine, chocolate
	Turnoffs: Garlic kisses, certain lubricants
Hearing	Turn-ons: Sexy talking, music, orgasmic moaning
	Turnoffs: Silence, television, offensive slang
Touch	Turn-ons: Lotions over sensitive areas, soaping each other, massage
	Turnoffs: Rough hands, touching only one area, beard stubble

Letting Passion Build. What a powerful turn-on as you build toward the apex. You are excited, your mate is excited with your excitement, and arousal has become a connecting experience. You are truly making love and enjoying your own unique pleasure in sensuality and intimacy.

Time Out: Discuss with your partner what are turn-ons and turnoffs in each of your senses: sight, smell, taste, hearing, and touch.

Stage 3: Apex

It takes a mature person to understand that the emotional center of the apex is not orgasm but a surrender to feelings and each other. The term *apex* is purposefully used to deemphasize chasing orgasms and to emphasize the deeper idea of abandonment to sensual arousal and closeness. Most often there will be that exciting climax, but there will be some times when an orgasm will not happen and yet an apex is achieved. Mature couples have often grown into this level of apex and enjoy the beauty of connection. As we grow older, we may not achieve an orgasm with every lovemaking cycle. After enjoyable love play, the couple may have reached the peak of their arousal for that session. They choose to progress into the *afterglow*. Souls have surrendered and joyful sexual experiences have been achieved, though no orgasm has occurred.

Focus on Pleasure Building. Stay in the moment with a growing focus on accenting what each partner is experiencing and needing. Some of this focus will be a personal, inner attention to building arousal. This does not exclude the mate but, almost like worship, our bodies and souls are reveling in the experience and taking in more and more. This is a special time of self as well as mutual sharing.

Greater Spiritual Connection. Look deeply into each other's eyes and get lost in the other and the sharing of passion. Lovemaking can make you more totally "naked" than any other mutual experience. Your emotions and your bodies are making three-dimensional music that is much more profound than the friction. Express your love with words and looks as you pair the union of body, soul, and spirit with climax.

Abandonment to Lovemaking; Surrender of Control and Climax. Think of what the word *abandon* means emotionally and physically. Maybe like a roller-coaster ride, you squeal and give in to powerful feelings, zooming down that steep slope. Or maybe you've experienced lifting your hands in worship and just giving in to God's presence and joy.

Apexes cannot be reached without surrendering control. It is interesting that many couples can create orgasms but not an apex because there are too many fears and walls to deep intimacy and trust. Let God help you surrender to Him and to each other on important nonsexual levels. This can create the foundation for sexual surrender and enjoying passionate climaxes—when you lose time and your body and feelings overwhelm the rational. What a precious gift to share with that lifetime lover—again and again with ever-increasing meaning and passion.

Stage 4: Afterglow

Mature lovers take care not to neglect this important stage, which may be three to five minutes or an hour. The afterglow may be even more important to the wife who has chosen to be vulnerable in physical and emotional ways. This is a time of affirmation to her that this was meaningful and real and loving. The husband also can enjoy and hook up his intimate emotions with his physical feelings—and even communicate more in this essential part of lovemaking.

Restabilizing, Cuddling, and Caressing. After the apex you need to catch your breath and come down physically and emotionally. This is the afterglow that is warmly intimate but less intense. Rather than jumping out of bed to clean up, hold each other and bask in the afterglow of intense connecting and shared surrender. Or, clean up and come back to bed for some minutes. Relax in the closeness and continue lovemaking in a more gentle and tender way. With your cuddling, include much eye contact and holding each other close. Your souls are connecting in this ongoing cycle of making love.

Affirmation, Reflection, and Basking. After being vulnerable, mates soak up praise and compliments. This can be a time of lovemaking that encourages compliments that may not come as quickly in the ordinary rush of life. Lay back and talk and affirm. Reflect and bask in the relationship, as well as in the events of the past moments, as you enrich your true lovemaking.

Feedback. Feedback can start the wheel rolling for the next lovemaking session: "Let's do that again," or "Could we make love Thursday morning?" It is better here to emphasize the positive, but laughing over the slipups, along with some future planning, is also in order. This is indeed an ongoing party, and we are enriching and preparing for the next festivity. Keep tuning in to all four aspects of atmosphere, arousal, apex, and after-glow—so the wheel of your love life experiences the ever-increasing passion God designed.

Time Out: Tell each other what parts of love-making you enjoy the most. Which stages of the Lovemaking Cycle are most appreciated by each of you?

Chapter 15

Vive la Différence:
Valuing Incompatibility

How fascinating that the wonderfully complex differences God brings to marriage give that companionship much of its richness and awesome fulfillment. One wonderful part about growing older is that we can more easily enjoy these differences. Many years of living life have pushed us to deal with and accept complexity. Shades of gray and seeming incompatibility are more comfortably embraced than if we were still in our thirties.

This chapter explores that granddaddy of all differences: the wonderful tensions and interesting dissimilarities of being male and female. But other differences play a part in great lovemaking too. Divergent personalities probably drive you crazy trying to blend the structured and spontaneous, reflective and extroverted, emotional and practical. As couples learn to accept and maximize each other's personality strengths, each lover will make unique and valuable contributions to the overall love-making. Other diversities like family background, previous experiences, and different thinking and communication styles must be understood and negotiated through to a more meaningful love life.

UNDERSTANDING MALE AND FEMALE DIFFERENCES

Lest we overemphasize the differences, another fascinating aspect in God's complex creation is that there is as much similarity between man and woman as there is in the three-person godhead. Males and females have more common emotions, needs, and attributes than they have differences. Each human being also contains aspects of both genders, and we can cultivate the best of both sexes.

In trying to understand and enjoy gender differences, remember that some are not God-designed distinctions, but cultural or learned. Don't panic because your spouse does not conform to the universal concepts of masculinity and femininity. Most people, especially as they grow older and wiser, blend characteristics from both lists.

MAKING LOVE TO YOUR WIFE

Men desperately want to be competent at all that they do. Making love can seem like a real setup, because your wife remains mysteriously complex. You think you've

CHARACTERISTICS OF MEN:

- Need to feel significant, admired, and respected, with sense of self-worth reinforced by affirmation and achievement; gain greater identity from what they do

- Take risks more easily (for example, no disability insurance)

- Are "one-track" and can be very focused on the opportunity of the moment (great strength and potential weakness, e.g., ballgame, completing a project, making love)

- Value self-sufficiency and can see life as a challenge and competition

- Desire to be competent and strong (can create defensiveness)

- Enjoy leading and providing (can lack flexibility and sensitivity to mate's desires)

- Less driven by feelings— can hold them in or lack the skills to express them; more left-brain and analytical, focused on a task

- Usually more hormonally driven (higher testosterone); tune in more visually to specific erotic cues and

CHARACTERISTICS OF WOMEN:

- Need to feel secure and have a comfortable nest as their safety and emotional needs are met; need to be attended to and made to feel special and adored

- Do not take risks as readily

- Can multitask easier and use both left and right brain (prone to distractions)

- Want to feel connected and included; gain greater identity from relationships

- See life as more of an interactive, cooperative community and desire connecting conversation and emotional connection

- Are better at asking connecting questions (can feel like interrogation to husband) and engaging in conversation

- Want to nurture and protect (strength and potential weakness with the mother-hen syndrome)

- Are freer in tuning in to and expressing emotions (can expect husband to understand or sense her feelings without communicating them) body parts, enjoy seeing their wife's body

- The eternal adolescent—childlike with curiosity and more immediate, playful enjoyment of sexuality (more prone to obsessive sexual behaviors)
- Are more predictable in what arouses them sexually

- Enjoy sensuality and tune in visually to the whole person as well as erogenous zones
- Desire romance and emotional affiliation in lovemaking
- Are unpredictable in sexual arousal, both mentally and physically

finally got it figured out, but then you bump your head again. Fortunately, maturity can help us live more easily and comfortably with these uncertainties as we understand, accept, and value our wives' mystique.

Uniquely Female

Try to walk in your wife's moccasins as you grow in understanding and skills. Granted, it will seem like she is speaking French while you speak German. Men can adapt and multitask some too. A husband can learn to speak a little French, especially if it will increase his ability to be a better lover.

Emotionally Connected Soul Mates. Women don't divorce sex as easily from the relational and emotional aspects as men can. A woman wants to feel cared about and emotionally connected before sexual activity can have appeal. For her, fun sex flows out of an intimate companionship that is emotionally close with plenty of physical affection and quality time together. I'm sorry, guys, but time and forethought are demanded here. The following formula helps to chart the difference between men and women:

MEN: *Physical* activity → connects the soul →
leads to *emotional* closeness
WOMEN: *Emotional* closeness → connects the soul →
opens the door to *physical* activity

Consistently Inconsistent. On one evening your wife may like oral stimulation of her clitoris or enjoy her breasts and nipples being caressed, and at another time she may not want that particular touch at all. Her body and reactions do not stay consistent, and you get confused. Your penis doesn't vary much, but she can change physically and emotionally by the hour—especially in these post-forty-five years.

Develop a series of strategies for making love. Become adept at smoothly switching gears from strategy A to strategy B to strategy E, depending on where your wife is in a given lovemaking session. Encourage her to say what she wants. Expect inconsistency and revel in your fast footwork and improvisational skills. She will love your spontaneous variety and your lack of irritability or pouting.

Vulnerable to Distraction. Women multitask better than men but are also more easily distracted by their environment and their inner attitudes and feelings. Husbands can falsely assume that their wives don't like sex as much as they do. When she is fatigued, fearful for her or her family's health, struggling with body image, or the bedroom is a mess, she may be unable to focus on her own arousal. Her desire to make love will be on the back burner. The wise husband minimizes distractions (e.g., bedroom picked up, phone calls made) and helps his wife begin to make love (romantic suggestion when leaving for work, sensual kissing in living room when he comes home) even before the bedroom.

Different Types of Initiating and Lovemaking. Sex is more purposeful, romantic, and intimate with a woman. It isn't the more immediate, hormonal surge that it can be with you. She will not think of sex as often as you do, but this is not from lack of desire. The timing must be appropriate, with plenty of love play as her body and emotions are "primed" and she is given the needed time for arousal. When lovemaking occurs and she can choose to get involved, she can respond with receptive desire (see Chapter 12) and a passionate enjoyment that create wonderful lovemaking. Husbands, as you age you will also become less testosterone-based and more intimacy-based.

| passionate | connecting | nurturing | duty |

Fig. 15.1 Types of Personal Involvement in Lovemaking

Maturity pushes us to rework our motivation and understanding of lovemaking. With women a varied continuum of reasons for lovemaking exist and most of them are very three-dimensional, with heart and intimacy more prominent than physical. *Duty* sex is an obligation out of guilt or pity with neither partner enjoying any real intimacy. *Nurturing* sex is honoring the higher need of one's partner but done willingly with various levels of participation. *Warm, slow,* and *tender* are the operative words in *connecting* sex, and often we have to be fifty to get this. *Passionate* may or may not include orgasms with more intensity and focus. Connecting sex may often move up and down the continuum between passionate and nurturing. Husbands, apart from lose-lose "pity" sex, allow your wife to nurture and connect in her unique and loving ways.

Husbands Becoming Passionate Lovers

Husbands, here are some tips for negotiating through the complexity of enjoying your masculinity and creating some great lovemaking.

Disputing Male Mythology. Probably the most prevalent male myth concerns the size of the penis. Do some self-talk and get over any feeling of inferiority. It's not the size or hardness that counts but how you enjoy sensuality and use it. Remember the old saying: "It's not the size of the boat, but the motion of the ocean." Another devastating myth is that men know all about sex and are always ready to go sexually. We have our knowledge and desire deficits just like women, but we often feel guilty admitting them.

Forget Your Obsessions. You have some fantasies and things you find sexy that your wife never will. She may never want to make love on an airplane or have anal sex. Don't wreck a great sex life by obsessing on what you think is the ultimate erotic adventure. You may also become obsessed with some part of her body that you wish were sexier, especially with aging. *Do not, and I repeat, do not, tell her these things.* Confess it to a buddy so he can tell you to grow up and learn true passion.

Be a Passionate Leader—Get a Ph.D. in "My Wife." Husbands, your wives' femininity is precious and unique.

Listen to her, observe her, try different things as you collect data, and be willing to make changes to please her. Most wives want husbands who are strong and confident and can provide unasked-for nurturing. Wives at times want to be "taken"—not in a demanding or abusive way but out of a passionate desire for their femininity from a self-confident husband. They want to be swept off their feet and fulfilled romantically.

MAKING LOVE TO YOUR HUSBAND

From the male perspective, there are few situations where sex doesn't add some spice and enhance the relationship. One wife stated that sex was her husband's solution to much of what he encountered in life. If he shot under par, he wanted to celebrate with sex; if he got frustrated or disappointed, he wanted to cheer up with sex. She related that the other day he swore it would help the flu. Making love is perhaps the primary means your husband uses to feel connected to you.

Some couples reading this book will find their situation reversed, with the wife having the higher urge for lovemaking. In the complexity of today's world, men can be overwhelmed and feel incompetent, sublimate their desire into accomplishing tasks, possess a fear of aging, or get their feelings hurt. Even if he doesn't fit across the board, many of these differences will still apply.

Uniquely Male

Some of your husband's actions and attitudes may stem from too many eggs in the sexual basket or a lack of three-dimensional intimacy. Much of his thinking and behavior, though, is due to the fact that you and he are wired differently.

Visually Specific and Genitally Focused with Mental Imagery. We're sure you've noticed how your husband is prone to zooming in on feminine parts. Research has shown that both men and women are aroused by visual stimulation, but they have different styles. A woman can drive by a cute male jogger, notice his strong physique, and immediately forget the visual stimulus. A man can see a female jogger and almost drive off the road trying to see in the rearview mirror what her breasts are like. If he sees you in panties, he doesn't stop there. He mentally takes one cue and tunes in to other sexual cues almost reflexively in his fantasy life.

Immediate and Quicker. Your husband has a tendency toward more immediate arousal and gratification. Wives may sometimes wonder if their husbands have remained sexual adolescents (even though it adds zest to their lovemaking). He thinks about sex a lot; he tends to forget consequences and jumps into pleasure, whether it means being late to a party or messing up her lipstick; he touches and grabs at what he likes; he loves the excitement of the moment and will savor lovemaking incidents to talk and think about later.

Predictable. What turns you on will vary constantly, but your husband is very predictable. If you initiate, appeal to him visually, or rub his penis, he usually gets excited. When you take risks and initiate something silly or different, it will seldom flop. Try to remember to include visual stimuli, some immediate gratification, and friction on specific locations. You will have a lot of power in a fun way sexually because he responds so predictably.

Wives Becoming Passionate Lovers

Every wife should be able to tune in to and enjoy the wonderful gift God has given her of femininity and sexual pleasure. Here are some tips for unleashing this tremendous capacity.

Disputing Female Mythology. Toxic myths abound about female sexuality. "Women aren't as sexual as men." "There are 'good girls' or 'bad girls.'" "Women so lack sexual self-awareness that when they say no, they actually mean yes." Wives, learn to dispute these misbeliefs and realize that some of them have arisen because men try to define sexual desire and female sexuality through male lenses.

Permission for Pleasure. Women can struggle with relaxing control and abandoning themselves to pleasure. This results from girls being taught psychologically to control sexual impulses and not to tune in to sexuality as readily. Even their genitals are more hidden and not grasped every time they urinate as men's are. Women also have a natural modesty that needs to be honored. You may need to intentionally tune in to your sexuality and make conscious choices to keep lovemaking on the front burner of your marriage:

1. Budget in and spend a certain amount of money each month on your sex life.

2. Every now and then wear a sexy piece of lingerie all day and allow its unusual feel to constantly remind you of sex, or use a special perfume that you have associated in your mind with making love.

3. Plan a sexual surprise at least once a month in which you try to blindside your husband in an arousing sexual way.

4. Create romantic sexual fantasies about your love life while driving in the car and share them with your mate at the end of your day.

Assertive Demands. You, as a woman, may enjoy a slower pace than your husband and need different types of touching. A basic part of turning yourself on is to assertively express your needs. Sex therapist Debra Taylor, in researching what women like most about sex, found that physical release was fourth behind physical closeness, emotional connection, and time together.[1] Sometimes you may want to cuddle and be held tight and have it lead nowhere. Become very direct in your requests; this will actually turn your husband on and allow yourself to experience more pleasure.

Passionate Power. You have tremendous power to arouse your husband. He desires and needs you. (*A crucial note:* Sometimes you won't turn him on. Don't assume he's too old, having an affair, or you're not attractive. Explore what is going on in his life. Persist through to healing and changes even if it takes professional help.) Fun flirting, playfully initiating sexual variety, and accentuating your femininity will increase the intimacy in your sexual companionship and is a definite win-win. Remember to honor your own personality, age, and femininity as you create your own brand of seductiveness. Just remember, you are tremendously alluring, and the most powerful attraction is your believing that.

To create fantastic lovemaking takes empathetic

understanding, loving acceptance, and a deep valuing of your incompatibility. Mates who have grown comfortable with the complementary nature of their person and gender let diversity create a rich and exciting lovemaking.

Chapter 16

Jump-Starting Your Love Life:
The Use of Sexual Aphrodisiacs

*T*he question is often asked: Do aphrodisiacs or magical sexual techniques really exist? Ginseng root, the Kama Sutra, hormones, Viagra, the Venus flutter, special herbs or teas—nothing has been proved to work universally. The Venus flutter was a spoof concocted on a television show to explain how one man, simultaneously married to thirteen women, kept them all sexually ecstatic. Sex therapists across the nation were reassuring clients that such a technique did not exist.

GO FOR THE NATURAL

Here's the good news about aphrodisiacs: Our gracious Creator has provided couples with many natural and revitalizing aphrodisiacs that can greatly enhance their lovemaking. We have organized these into five general categories: emotional, practical, relational, sensual, and behavioral.

1. Emotional Aphrodisiacs

Emotionally Open and Passionate. An ancient Greek philosopher stated that "the passions are the winds that fill the sails of our souls." Expressing feelings and becoming emotionally passionate sometimes become more subdued in adulthood and older age—as we have learned to moderate our feelings. (Also, some personalities and men in general naturally express fewer feelings and will have to choose to let go.) If a quality of maturity is not caring so much what others think, then let the feelings roll.

Take a ride on the wild side of feelings and bring them back into your bedroom. What a fun discipline to practice. Dance joyously at a wedding as you do the hokeypokey; ride a roller coaster screaming with your mouth wide open; jump into a cold lake on a hot summer day. Risk stronger feelings in your love life, and you will be amazed at how your partner is turned on by a passionate person.

Time Out: A marvelous aphrodisiac is that God has given us imaginations to create mental and emotional sexual fantasies. Sit quietly a minute and imagine a romantic sexual encounter with your mate. Share this with him/her at the end of your day.

Mysteriously Romantic. Our God is a God of mystery, romance, adventure, and endlessly creative variety. The prophet Jeremiah writes in amazement, "His compassions never fail. They are new every morning" (Lam. 3:22–23 NIV). Each day we can create a *new* relationship with our Creator—and also with our human lover and mate.

It is amazing how lovers come up with the unusual when unleashing their romantic side and planning erotic surprises. One husband arranged a complete weekend, from talking to his wife's boss about picking her up from work early, to sexy lingerie and her bags packed, to a surprise spot (he had scouted it out) they had never been to.

Erotically Adored. Years ago when I [Doug] started dating my Cathy, had you asked me one of the things that was so appealing about her, I would have quickly responded, "She totally adores me." I desired and valued from a human partner what God feels for those He loves. "I have summoned you by name; you are mine" (Isa. 43:1 NIV).

A critical aspect of erotically adoring someone is unconditional acceptance, as a person can come to be naked and exposed physically and emotionally and still feel comfortable. What a turn-on for celebrating sex after fifty. Looking through the eyes of love creates an adoration of the person that transcends wrinkles, cellulite, and human foibles. One of my friends relates that at parties he will look across the room and wink at his wife of many years. She will light up because he has so constantly told her, "You are the most attractive woman here, and I'm lucky to have you." Now just the wink conveys that message of adoration.

2. Practical Aphrodisiacs

Sexual Goal Setting. Some couples fear that consciously making decisions and setting goals around their love life will stunt the passion and spontaneity. Goal setting is simply a means to an end and doesn't have to dampen excitement and creativity. Sexual goals involve more than increasing sexual frequency and should begin with the quality of your lovemaking and the quality of your intimate companionship. Goals may include reading at least a chapter a month in a book on sex, each mate initiating one new technique or idea as a contribution to creativity and variety, or scheduling regular vacation times.

Physically Fit and Rested. Good health and physical fitness are marvelous aphrodisiacs. Being rested revitalizes attitudes and makes sexual activity more appealing. Getting the body in shape with long walks or other forms of exercise enhances sex with improved blood flow and muscle tone. Making vigorous love affirms your sense of physical well-being. As we age, this aphrodisiac may need more intentional work as we work through illnesses and sleeplessness.

3. Relational Aphrodisiacs

Prioritizing the Present. A husband complained that his wife was so distracted she had asked if the clothes were in the dryer at the height of their lovemaking. She stated he wasn't much better. Last night at a tender moment, he had exclaimed those endearing words, "Oh, no; my mom's visit starts tomorrow." They were praying that God would help them both bring their hearts, minds, and bodies into the bedroom to mutually enjoy their love life.

An early church father, Jean Pierre de Cassaude, said it beautifully as he encouraged every Christian to carefully honor "the sacrament of the present moment." It is exciting and tremendously romantic to be fully present and available to another person—no distractions or preoccupations. Just the two of you there in that moment.

Quantity Time. So often in marriage, we try to find those small windows of quality time to balance out too many commitments or a lack of priority on connecting. Intimacy withers if all that is given is small doses of quality time. Real companions spend time together and become best friends. Slowing down in later years doesn't guarantee this. Most of us know older couples who have created totally separate lives. Great lovemaking depends on companions who grow closer with shared intimacies. Creating fun sexual and nonsexual traditions will take some quantity, not just quality, time—and intentional choices to be together as best friends.

Traditions and History. The mature years have an advantage in an important aspect of intimate relationships. Deep, consistent love is built on knowing someone over time. It's repeating activities and building a history together over the years as events take on deeper meaning and become traditions. Building up a *shared history with fun traditions* can be a tremendous aphrodisiac. Favorite positions, shared memories and fantasies, and tender touches on familiar bodies take hours and years to grow.

4. Sensual Aphrodisiacs

The Bedroom. The bedroom will be the primary love nest with special mood-setting qualities. Live flowers, mood lighting or candles, sensuous linens, a comfortable mattress, plenty of pillows, and the ability to control the temperature are sexual enhancements. You are pairing in your mind the bedroom with fun, sensual, erotic experiences. Just walking into the bedroom should create a different mood. Do some brainstorming as you spice it up.

Props. The words *sex toys* conjure up the idea of chasing a sexual rush versus truly making love. We have deliberately chosen the word *props* because celebrating sex after fifty can definitely utilize some strategic aids (much more comprehensive than sex toys) in comfortably and passionately enjoying each other. Candles, music, lotions, and lingerie stimulate ambience and help mature lovers enjoy aging bodies. Perhaps the most important props are pillows. Pillows are great to lean against in positions of pleasuring and intercourse. They help make the bed the playground it should be. Purchase various shapes and sizes, and use them to support necks (tube pillow), backs (large), or prop up buttocks (bed pillow).

Couples sometimes worry that certain props like vibrators may create artificial or wrongful arousal, and will detract from their natural lovemaking. God gave us imaginations and the ability to be romantic in order to create and enjoy various means of enticing and playing with our mates. Props simply enhance experiences and sensations and should (1) remain playfully in perspective and never become an obsessive fetish, (2) not detract from your vulnerability and respect, because arousal is dependent on feeling safe and inviting true passion and connection in all three dimensions of body, soul, and spirit, and (3) never invite anyone else into your bedroom, as pornography does.

Some husbands worry that a vibrator will create sensations that cannot be duplicated by him in creating orgasms, and may become addictive. I have not seen addiction but can understand the couple who do not wish to become dependent on a vibrator to create a climax for the wife. But for some women, a vibrator can enhance their ability to achieve an orgasm and seems very appropriate. They also are great for aching muscles and full body massage.

5. Behavioral Aphrodisiacs

Self-Nurture. Take a leisurely bath and indulge in other sensual delights at the end of a tiring day—it is a great aphrodisiac and tunes you in to your own body. In the midst of all your demands, you must learn to be self-nurturing. It will keep you sexier.

Creative Initiating. Use a special cologne that you have associated in your mind with making love, and wear it on the evening or the day you anticipate sexual activity.

Sexual Flooding. Many husbands dream about being ravished by so much sex they couldn't stand more. At a time when you are feeling relaxed, rested, and free for activity—tell your mate that he is free to initiate sex whenever he desires on a given day. Unleash a flood of sexual activity. What an aphrodisiac, as both mates enjoy this playful interaction and create for each other romantic, sensuous pleasure.

The Art of Kissing. Women especially enjoy variety in kissing, and the mouth can be extremely sensuous.

Lightly kiss all over her face and body, keeping lips soft and gentle, like a butterfly flitting about. Practice a gentle sucking motion on your wife's nipples, her fingers or toes, her neck, or her lower lip. There is something passionate and intimate about sharing mouths and tongues. Long, exciting kisses, where you have to come up for breath, make kissing an arousing, drawn-out affair.

Exaggerated Climaxes. Focus on your arousal and take time to build your sexual excitement. At the point of climax, release the tension with gusto and force. Encourage each other to make loud noises, expressions of pleasure, and exaggerate the muscle spasms. This is not about aging bodies performing but is rather a playful acting out of strong release, which can increase the fun and excitement of lovemaking for both of you.

As you think back over the many aphrodisiacs and begin applying them, ponder this saying from the Talmud, the Jewish teachings on the first five books of Scripture: "God will hold us accountable for every permitted pleasure that we forfeit." This, of all eras of the life span, can be a time of creative, playful, and passionately intimate lovemaking.

Chapter 17

Magic Fingers:
Sensuous Massage and
Mutual Pleasuring

Do you want to feel more in love and grow old graciously together as lovers? Then make the time to touch, massage, and pleasure each other's bodies (and souls). Massage has been shown to have profound effects on the one giving the massage as well as the person receiving. With touch the body releases oxytocin, a peptide secreted in the brain, which sensitizes the skin, increases sexual receptivity, and promotes bonding between lovers. Touch also reduces stress, blood pressure goes down, aging muscles and arthritic joints are soothed, and a relaxed and close, nurturing atmosphere is encouraged.

SETTING THE STAGE FOR MASSAGE

There really are few preparations or necessary items other than some oil or lotion and a quiet, warm place to lie during the massage.

Oils and Lotions

Natural oils like coconut, sesame, safflower, almond, soy, or avocado work well. Some natural oils like olive, peanut, or corn oil can be too thick and don't spread or absorb as easily. Lotions dry out quicker, but the scent and texture can be sensual. Be sure to warm both the oil and your hands before applying. Use only enough oil or lotion so the hands move smoothly over the skin.

Table, Mat, or Bed

A bed does not work well for some massage because it is too soft and will prevent firm, even pressure. If you have a table that comes to your upper thigh, find a mat or a piece of foam rubber or use blankets and towels to cover it. Beds work well for many types of sensual and sexual pleasuring.

Ambience

Adjust the thermostat, soften the lighting, light candles, and create a relaxing, sensuous atmosphere. Be sure to remove your jewelry and warm your hands. You may want to buy a flannel sheet to drape the parts of the body you are not massaging. Keep towels (or pillows) handy to roll up under the neck or other areas that need support.

BASIC TECHNIQUES OF MASSAGE

Massage is not complex. Basic techniques include: (1) the fundamental movements with rhythms and pressure, and (2) types of strokes and touch.

Movements

Rhythms. A soothing and sensuous massage should maintain a smooth and even rhythm with strokes that flow into one another. It should have a relaxing, almost hypnotic effect. One technique for accomplishing this is trying to always have at least one hand on the body at all times.

Pressure. A common mistake is thinking that massage, to be effective, must always be firm. Sometimes a light stroke or a hand lying on a body part will start nerves and skin tingling and will feel very sensuous. If there is a problem with sensitivity or ticklishness, try a firmer touch. If that doesn't work, move on to a less ticklish part; often you can come back later.

Stroking and Passive Touching

You will use stroking the most in your massage as you glide your hands over the skin with modified pressure. Remember the importance of a steady rhythm in which you vary the pressure and speed of the movements. Here are some variations of stroking motions and passive touching:

Fan Stroking. Start with your hands together and move them upward, applying pressure with palms and heels as you lean in to stroke. Maintain gentle pressure as you mold your hands to the body and slide them up the abdomen and lower back. Fan your hands out and lessen pressure as you glide them down and around the sides. With light pressure, move hands back into position to begin the stroke again.

Alternate Stroking. One hand strokes upward while the other hand glides downward in alternating motions—the upward stroke can be firmer as you vary pressure.

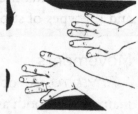

Thumb Stroking. Apply pressure on an area with the thumbs in small, firm circular movements, or slowly move them up and down the spine with firm, even pressure.

Brush Stroking. With fingertips or entire hand, sensitize the skin by *very* lightly brushing an area of the body. This stroke is often used at the end of massaging a given part of the body.

Passive Touching. You don't always have to be actively massaging a body area. Simply placing a hand on a spot as the partner's body feels the warmth or pressure (if applied) really feels good as tissue is stimulated by the passive touch. Passive touch also includes pulling or rotating a part of the body to loosen up and exercise joints without actively stroking.

1. Pressure. Place your hands over the tailbone area and leave them there lightly for thirty seconds—now lean into your hands with pressure but no movement.

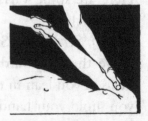

2. Lifting, pulling, and rotating. Lift your partner's arm up and down several times and gently pull up on it; now slowly rotate it in a circular motion several times. Hold it a few seconds and then lay it down.

SENSUOUS MASSAGE FOR SPECIFIC AREAS OF THE BODY

Massaging all areas of the body can bring tension release and sensuous pleasure to your mate with massage. We have included a few examples, but use your creativity as you improvise and create your own types of touching and sequences on various areas of the body. After massaging an area, hold your hands there a few seconds to seal the nurturing of that part.

Foot Massage

Stroking. Do one foot at a time. Grasp it firmly as you stroke it from ankle to heel and down the arch to

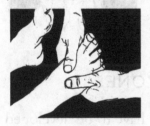

the toes. Hold the foot with both hands and do thumb strokes on the back of foot—stroke between the tendons and up and over arch and around the base of the ankle.

Passive Touching. Grasp the ankle and with the other hand manipulate the foot. Hold the foot and apply pressure with your thumbs at various points of the arch.

Chest and Neck Massage

Fan Stroking. Position yourself behind your partner's head and place your hands below the collarbone.

Press down the chest, then fan across the pectoral muscles to the shoulders and bring fingers with pressure up the back of the shoulders and neck and back to the original place. Repeat.

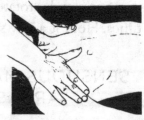

Face Massage

Stroking with Fingertips. Do small circles with both hands using fingertips on the temples, jaw, base of skull, and carefully around the eyes and forehead.

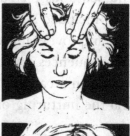

Passive Touching. With your hands cupping your partner's face, gently press on the temple area. Rest your fingertips on the eyes. Press on the forehead with one hand over the other.

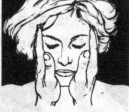

EROGENOUS ZONES

Sensuality and sensitivity to touch have to be developed and connected to your lovemaking. Our erogenous zones are more alike than different, whether we are male or female, overweight or underweight, young or old. But some individuals will experience more sensitivity and arousal from certain erogenous spots than from others. These may also change over time. The erogenous areas can be divided into three levels according to their sensitivity in producing sensual and sexual arousal.

Level Three

This level includes the entire body with its skin and nerve endings. Level three erogenous zones such as the feet or back are the focus of most massages. Sensate focus is a structured exercise for engaging in full-body massage.

Sensate Focus
(for Level Three Zone)

Sensate focus is a great way to develop the art of sensual touching and is often a prescribed part of sex therapy because it takes the focus off performing and places it on mutual sharing and sensuality. In this exercise, both partners are nude with thirty minutes blocked out as each takes the role of giver/toucher (15 minutes) and receiver/touchee (15 minutes).

The Active Toucher. The active mate touches the passive partner in ways that feel good to the toucher. This touching is oriented toward individual pleasure, sensuality, and enjoyment of the mate's body. There are no performance needs. Experiment with a variety of touches and strokes on any area other than the genitals and breasts. It is often helpful to start with the touchee lying on the stomach. Begin at the top of the head and slowly work your way down to the feet. Have the passive partner roll over, and work from the feet to the head.

The Passive Touchee. The touchee lies passively and allows the active partner to touch the body. Often the touches that pleasure the active toucher give stimulation and pleasure to the passive mate too. The passive partner can increase self-awareness by noticing which areas and types of touching give the greatest pleasure. You can ask for these to be repeated while making love at a different time. The touchee is also learning about the lover—what kind of touching and strokes the toucher usually enjoys to give and receive.

Level Two

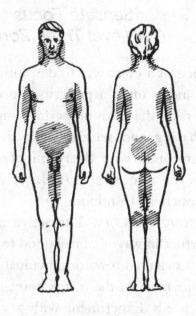

Fig. 17.1.
Level two
erogenous zones
[silhouette of front
of male and back
of female]

This level includes parts of the body that are normally stimulated during foreplay or intercourse. If you desire to be a great lover, become familiar with these areas of your partner's body. Take fingertips or mouth and tongue and stimulate the sensory nerve endings as you discover where more pleasurable feelings lie: (1) the back of the knees, (2) the inner thighs, (3) the armpits and breast area, (4) the abdomen area and the navel, (5) the small of the back and buttocks, (6) the neck from back to front, (7) the palms of the hands and bottoms of the feet, (8) the face, especially the (9) eyelids, (10) the edges of the nose over the sinus cavities, (11) the temples, and (12) the mouth and tongue. These areas are rich in sensory nerve endings and can be a sensual treat, rather than immediately focusing in on level one zones.

Level One

The most sensitive and sexually stimulating erogenous zones are the nipples and the genitals. Don't neglect the nipples as a favorite spot of both men and women for stimulating sexual excitement. The nerve endings are especially sensitive and connected to sexual arousal. The genitals most directly stimulate sexual arousal, and the last section of this chapter carefully explores this aspect of lovemaking.

Mutual Pleasuring (Levels One and Two Erogenous Zones)

Pleasure is an interesting word. Somehow it almost does not seem to fit within Christian values. It feels selfish and self-centered. The truth is that enjoying genital pleasuring that is slow and bonding without pressure and demands is critical to a truly intimate, nurturing, and exciting sex life. You need to be able to make love for half an hour to a couple of hours at a time.

Position for Pleasuring: Sitting with Back to Chest. This relaxing position lends itself to non-demanding body and genital pleasuring of various kinds. Aging muscles may need to strategically use pillows or the back of the bed to prop up and get comfortable.

This position has the pleasuree sitting comfortably

between the legs of the pleasurer, leaning back against his or her chest to be cuddled and pleasured. The hands of the pleasurer have access to the chest and genitals of the partner. The pleasurer can be propped up against the back of the bed for comfort. An important part of non-demanding pleasuring is feeling close and connected as you sensuously give pleasure and enjoy your mate's body.

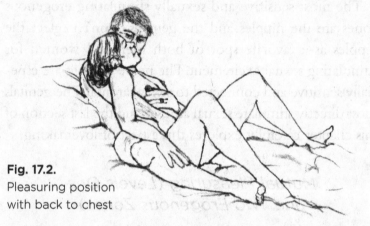

Fig. 17.2.
Pleasuring position
with back to chest

Use your imagination to overcome size and weight differences. For example, if the husband is taller or heavier, then let him scoot down and pleasure his head, shoulders, and nipples. Then, the wife can let him be comfortably propped up sitting and she can sensuously cuddle in, with her breasts against his side as she pleasures his genitals. The goal is intimate touch and skin-to-skin closeness.

NURTURING THROUGH ORGASMS

George had a higher desire for sexual activity than Helen did. She explained that it wasn't that she didn't like sex or have a desire to make love. She just did not want to become actively involved on some evenings when she was fatigued. The following technique revolutionized their sex life. At least once a week, she pleasured him to an orgasm without her active participation.

She would slip off her nightgown and gently hold his testicles while he stroked himself to a climax. She did not mind his fondling her breasts, and she appreciated the pleasure she brought him even with the minimal involvement. Sometimes she would place her hand over his and in other small ways would be supportive. She snuggled close to him and afterward used a warm washcloth to help him clean up. Often that type of sexual activity would not take more than ten minutes, but he found it nurturing and fulfilling. They still felt like they were making love.

For other couples, the husband may pleasure his wife when he is not in the mood or feels tired. Nurturing through orgasm can be a loving compromise in a sexual partnership.

THE PLEASURE OF ORAL STIMULATION

In the same way that kissing and intimately sharing mouths brings erotic arousal and intimate bonding, oral stimulation of the genitals can build trust and be exciting for mates. A quick bath and good hygiene are crucial for this genital pleasuring. Don't worry about his climaxing in your mouth—you as wife are assertive and can ask for what you do and don't want. Actively share your needs and sensibilities.

The Song of Solomon implies oral sex with "browsing among the lilies," but this does not make it right for you. You as mates will have to sort and pray through various behaviors as you choose what to include in your repertoire of lovemaking. Never make your mate feel guilty or inhibited because he or she does not feel comfortable with a given behavior. The object is to be playful, lovingly connected, and creatively varied.

Trusting your genitals to your mate's mouth is warmly intimate and symbolic. Husbands are very protective of the penis and testicles. To allow the partner complete access is an important commitment, as they feel very vulnerable and in turn arousingly close. Wives have sometimes bought into the notion that somehow they are dirty down there, or they have left their genitals as an unknown area. To have the husband intimately scrutinizing and enjoying this part of the body takes special trust and openness.

Here are a few suggestions for wife and husband to enhance this variety of genital pleasuring:

Wife, use your lips as buffers for your teeth in order to prevent damage to sensitive tissue. Use tongue and mouth to tease the head of the penis, as you manually stroke the shaft of the penis and create firmer stimulation. Allow your mouth to create a vacuum effect—the stronger the sucking action, the more pleasurable feelings produced. The head of the penis is the most sensitive part—don't worry about trying to take more of the penis in your mouth.

Husband, tease with your tongue as you flick it lightly over the vulval area. Kiss and gently suck the entire area.

If your tongue gets tired, hold it firm and create rubbing sensations by moving your entire head from side to side. You can also create sucking motions with your mouth over the clitoris to produce a climax. Remember, the clitoris can be very sensitive. Keep teeth covered and employ variety until she actively approaches an orgasm.

Oral sex can be interspersed with other types of genital pleasuring in a nondemanding, emotionally connecting manner. It can be more exciting at times if combined with simultaneous manual stimulation. While enjoying oral sex, you can keep your hands active, too, as the clitoris is sucked or the penis and testicles are stroked, fingers are inserted into the vagina, or the back and chest is caressed, the buttocks are massaged, and the skin is teased.

Keep balanced in your lovemaking, and don't just focus on intercourse and orgasm. Always keep in mind that the platform for great sex is your wonderful marital companionship—all kinds of touch will nurture your love in amazing ways.

Chapter 18

Ooh La La!:
Creative Intercourse and Lovemaking

$\mathcal{A}$ new client opened up a session by saying there were over four hundred positions of intercourse and he wanted to learn them all. Actually, there are only about eight basic types, with further variations like woman on top winking her right eye, but isn't it great to be older? Learning twenty, much less four hundred positions, has no appeal to us. We're more like the wife who wanted a position or two that would minimize her husband's belly, be comfortable for her arthritis, and hit her G-spot.

In reality, unleashing a little creativity, feeding your enjoyment of variety, risking something new—then relaxing in the tried and true, and being sensuous lovers are the vital components of fun intercourse. You control the candlelight, music, lotions, lubrication, and ambience as you allow intercourse and various positions to be interspersed throughout your lovemaking. Each position will offer a variety of ways to stimulate, touch, and take pleasure from each other's body in heartfelt ways.

ENHANCING INTERCOURSE

You as a couple can help intercourse provide arousing connection, meet different needs, and enhance your lovemaking. Here are some important considerations:

1. Are you comfortably supported so muscles don't grow weary and neither partner feels squashed or smothered? Utilize a lot of pillows. Are you positioned with enough leverage to create easy thrusting movements so that husband or wife or both can produce exciting friction?

2. Does the position allow for good penetration—not too deep or too shallow—with the penis, and is it hitting the right spots in the vagina or on the penis? The G-spot is about a half inch into the vagina at twelve o'clock (toward the navel). Kegel exercises (see Chapter 3) can help increase arousal for both husband and wife.

3. Are props convenient to the lovemaking: pillows, lubrication, tissues, candles, lotions, and other needed/ enjoyed items?

4. Is there visual contact and is it arousing and intimate—with the husband and wife enjoying each other's genitals and body, and both appreciating eye-to-eye connection?

5. Does the position allow manual or oral contact with the body, breasts, or genitals? Can you kiss, cuddle, and caress—stroke the scrotum or clitoris while thrusting?

Does it allow either partner to take a more initiating role as desired to produce arousal?

You know the old saying that "practice makes perfect." First, do some preliminary learning with the book beside you as you learn a new position and try it out. Second, incorporate the new position into your lovemaking over the next week or two as you truly make it yours. Be playful and creative as you make up some of your own variations to try. Also practice shifting into a new position from an existing position without removing the penis. This creates fun moves and erotic love play.

POSITIONS OF INTERCOURSE

The next section of this chapter develops some basic intercourse positions. Learn what fits you two, but do be creative and try some new positions as you adapt them to your celebration of sex after fifty. Consider how certain positions could enhance your lovemaking, as well as fit within your unique limitations in the aging process. Men and women vary in physical and psychological arousal and will have differing preferences about what is exciting to them. Allow intercourse to enrich your love life as your hands and mouth keep actively caressing and stroking throughout the process of soulful body-to-body connection. Remember that you as unique lovers take these neutral techniques and give them playful, creative sensuality.

Wife-on-Top Kneeling

The wife-on-top positions are favorites for several reasons. For the husband who has a bad back or knees, this position takes the pressure off and allows his wife to be the active participant. It is also the needed position for a couple with disabilities who want to press into the vagina the flaccid penis of the husband. The positions are visually very arousing to the male, and the female is more in control of her own stimulation. This also allows her to control the depth of penetration, which is important in the postmenopausal vagina that may have less padding. Many women find being on top positions the vagina and clitoris to achieve orgasm more readily during intercourse. The husband's hands are also nicely placed to stimulate the clitoris as needed.

Fig. 18.1.
Wife-on-Top

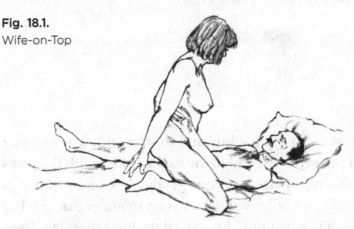

The wife kneels while she straddles her husband with a 90-degree upright stance with bouncing motions or a 45-degree forward tilt with weight on arms or forearms propped on pillows. It is also pleasurable to simply let the erect penis lie on his stomach and, with proper lubrication, rub the clitoral area back and forth with a rocking motion across the hard penis without vaginal penetration.

Husband-on-Top Legs Straddling

This has often been called the missionary position because, according to legend, the Hawaiians did not employ this position. They were surprised to discover that the missionaries to their land used it exclusively. It may be an apocryphal story, but this standard position is often thought of as uncreative or elementary. Actually, it is pleasurable in various ways. It allows deep penetration, active thrusting by the husband, wife stimulating her clitoris, and a total body hug with much eye-to-eye lovemaking.

Fig. 18.2.
Husband-on-Top Legs Straddling

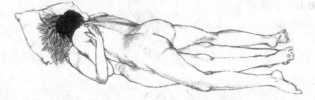

It is easier for the husband to start with legs together and the penis inserted in the vagina. Now, with the penis remaining inserted, he can gently shift one of his legs outside one of his wife's legs as he straddles that leg. For different sensations, he can shift his other leg from between to outside as he straddles with both legs outside his wife's legs. This allows his wife to clamp or scissor her legs together and produce greater friction on the penis in her vagina, and the husband can raise up on his knees and elbows to relieve any excess pressure on his wife. Relax in intercourse hugs or roll over into a side or woman-on-top position (when husband's legs are inside wife's or straddling her one leg).

Wife Straddling Husband's Leg

Couples enjoy side-by-side positions because bodies are comfortably close and facing each other for cuddling and kissing. Bodies are well supported, and both partners can control and contribute to coital thrusting while they caress and stroke.

Fig. 18.3.
Wife Straddling Husband's Leg

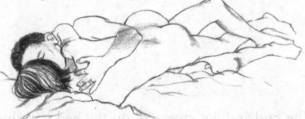

The husband lies comfortably on his side, with his bottom leg extended straight, his other leg bent at the knee, and his foot on the bed. The wife lies on her side and straddles the top bent leg, with her lower leg between his legs and her top leg thrown over his torso. Guiding the penis to the vagina will often take both partners' cooperation. Again, pillows under heads or sides increase comfort.

Crosswise Scissoring Wife's Leg

This crosswise position can become a favorite with hands free to use the penis as a wand to stimulate the clitoris like a vibrator. Or, while the husband is thrusting, the wife can caress his testicles or scissor two of her fingers around his thrusting penis to increase stimulation. The husband can maneuver his body (collapsing the straight + into a collapsed cross X), while keeping the penis in the vagina so that he is able to nibble at her breasts and enjoy kissing, too—with hand caressing of tummy and thighs.

Fig. 18.4.
Crosswise Scissors

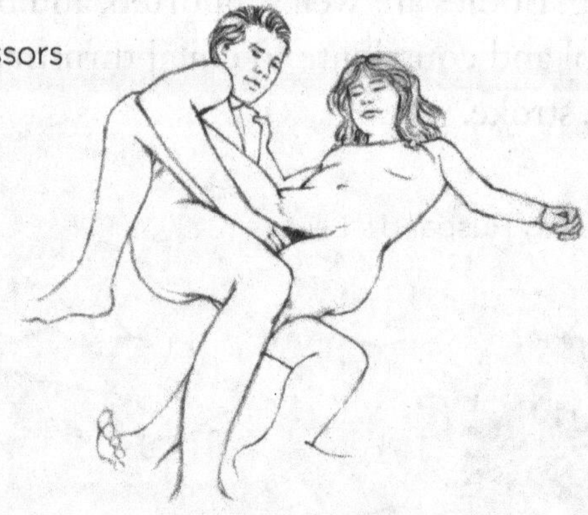

The husband lies crosswise on the bed with his head to the wife's right, and she lies on her back. This time the wife's right leg is propped over her husband's thighs, and her left leg is scissored between her husband's legs. She can raise her leg so her husband's elbow is around her ankle. If the husband is left-handed, he scissors her right leg, placing his head on her left side to allow manipulation of penis.

From the scissor position, the couple can maneuver into the rear-entry spoons position without withdrawing the penis. The wife rolls onto her side with her back toward the husband. The husband gently unscissors her leg, then slides his legs so they are behind hers in a spoon position as he thrusts against her buttocks. Both the scissors and spoons positions make less demand on muscles and joints—great positions for aging bodies or for a break from more active love play to massage and caress.

Rear-Entry as Spoons

The spoons position allows the husband to give his wife a wonderful back and neck massage while thrusting—which can be as gentle or vigorous as desired. There is a pressure point at the lower back/tailbone that the husband can reach with his thumbs for arousal.

Fig. 18.5.

Rear-entry Spoons

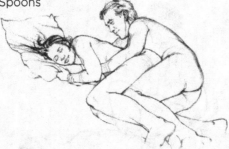

The husband faces his wife's back, like two spoons cradling. The penis can be inserted with the husband separating legs and outer vulval lips, while the wife guides the penis into the vagina. Male pelvic thrusting bumps softly against her buttocks as the penis stimulates the front of the vagina and the G-spot. The husband can enjoy caressing his wife's stomach and breasts and stimulating her clitoris with his free hand.

Wife on the Edge

This position can be great for men with knee replacements, especially if the bed is high enough. The bed is a comfortable object for the wife to be on the edge of, but don't limit creativity. Dining room tables and kitchen counters are higher, and easy chairs work well if kneeling. Many beds are too low and pillows will be needed or the man will need to lower his body. This position is very visually stimulating to the husband: He can observe the vulval area and the penis thrusting in and out. It is exciting to the wife: She can observe her partner's arousal by her body as well as experience her own visual excitement. Her vagina and clitoris can receive excellent friction in this position.

Fig. 18.6.
Wife on Edge

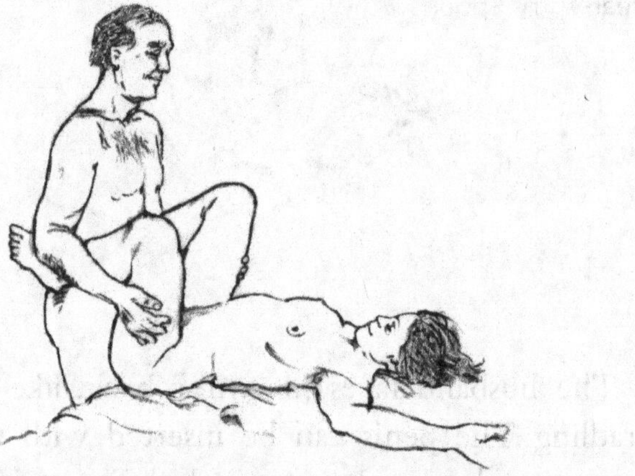

The wife is positioned at the edge of the bed or counter. Her legs are around her husband's torso, resting comfortably on his thighs, with his arms supporting and clamping her legs to his body. The husband kneels or stands, depending on the height of the object the wife is on, so his penis is accessible to her vagina. He has an easy thrusting motion, and the wife may not be fully reclined but propped up on the pillows of an easy chair and have access to stroking and caressing herself and her husband. The wife-on-the-edge position lends itself to all rooms of the house and provides some fun variation because it can be enjoyed without total removal or wrinkling of clothes.

As we age we need to create our own variations and

adapt positions to our bodies and our limitations. Be curious and experimental as you take the risks to try new positions, and learn them well enough that they become comfortable. Truly frolic and laugh and love as you enjoy making intercourse a fun part of your sex life.

CREATIVE LOVEMAKING

Making love is much more than just getting nude or rushing into intercourse. Wise lovers know how to incorporate variety into their intimate passion. Remember the importance of uninterrupted privacy, effective timing, a sensual setting, and keeping an open invitation to make love.

1. Gourmet Marathon

Perhaps the most precious gift mates can give each other is time. Never believe that because you are over fifty that a couple of hours in bed is beyond your capacity. With gourmet lovemaking, all five senses are emphasized with much creative variety. Lovers can vary the tempo from intense to languid. Intercourse and orgasms will be included at various times along the way, but intimate connecting of all kinds is the course du jour.

2. Quick Encounter

God created us with nerve endings, an important feeling center in our brain called the amygdala, and an enjoyment of adventure and romance. No wonder mates enjoy the spontaneous fun of sexual quickies. To indulge in immediate arousal and gratification is hilarious and uninhibited—that spontaneous romp and unexpected climax in the daily routine.

3. Playful Romp

Great lovers know how to revel in their child-ego state. Children are so fascinating as everything becomes a toy or a game, with playful romps the norm. Adults forget how to frolic and tickle and squeal with delight. Props can be fun, like a shower and soaping each other up or feathers or food or Crisco oil with lighthearted laughter and simple fun.

4. Erotic Volcano

It is fun to deliberately build passionate erotic arousal and create intense orgasmic feelings—either one partner at a time or somewhat mutually. Some of this buildup is having enough prelude and teasing, erotic setup. Then it is focusing in on personal arousal and allowing the sexual tension to increase with rapid friction as you approach orgasm, and then back off, enjoying this plateau phase. (*Note:* The partner giving the pleasure increases the mate's arousal by mirroring his or her approaching climax with empathetic groans of pleasure, tense muscles, and heavier breathing.) Finally, hang on the edge with muscles tense and holding your breath—and then truly abandon your inhibitions and surrender to the explosion.

5. Fantasy Enrichment

Remember that our mind, with its imagination and mental imagery, is the most crucial sexual organ for great lovemaking. We create a whole depository of sexual memories over the years that can be very stimulating and bonding. The reminders can come in various ways, like sitting together and reminiscing about special times together. Lovers need to occasionally act out that fantasy with the Hawaiian shirt and the smell of suntan lotion on a dreary January evening. The mind and emotions can so marvelously pull us out of the ordinary and into the magic world of imagination and romance.

6. Connecting Companionship

Sometimes sex just needs to be warmly comfortable. Your mutually favorite position and the old tried-and-true caresses fit the bill. Massaging tender and intimate areas like face and tummy—giving each other a full-body intercourse hug fills those inner longings. It may get a little vigorous or it may stay quite gentle with those slow hands. Best friends who love to laugh and be together—even if they weren't lovers—and the sexual connecting just make it more special.

In passionately intimate marriages, erotic sexuality and lovemaking permeate the atmosphere and relationship. I [Doug] am so touched when I see that couple in their eighties who are still sexual and seductive with inviting lover-looks and touches.

Chapter 19

God's Sexual Emergency Room:
Healing Relational Wounds

*O*ver the years, boomers have had to come to grips with the basic fact that it's a broken world and humans make mistakes. Sin and stupidity abound, and we could become jaded and cynical with no interest in risking intimacy. Our wounds extend back into childhood, and unfortunately, every major transition can resurrect many of these old hurts and impediments. We don't want to waste a lot of time and energy refusing to resolve these wounds.

Fortunately, after Adam and Eve sinned and relationships started spiraling down, our loving Creator gave us skills for healing damaged or threatened intimacy. So when we're broken and hurting, especially sexually, we can come to God's emergency room. This ER is equipped with the healing instruments for correcting our distorted situations and helping us get back into God's love and light and wisdom. *Maturity masters these critical skills for healing intimacy.* Which of these do you need to work on to deepen your intimacy and create a true celebration of lovemaking?

CONFRONTING

The apostle Paul told Timothy that he should learn to "correct, rebuke and encourage—with great patience and careful instruction" (2 Tim. 4:2 NIV). We need to take on the qualities of Christ, who "is able to deal gently with those who are ignorant and are going astray" (Heb. 5:2 NIV). We all know that there is a lot of sin and immaturity in all of our lives. Being over fifty doesn't give us exemptions from marital difficulties, broken sexuality, poor boundaries, or real skill deficits. We can help each other conform to God's guidelines through skillful confrontation—through assertively and honestly surfacing and dealing with issues and feelings.

A hurting, motivated wife came for counseling and stated she had faithfully practiced submission, hoping to help her husband make some needed changes. I [Doug] replied that submission would create an atmosphere in which change could take place, but that submission was not God's tool for accomplishing change. Confrontation was that needed skill. She needed to get in her husband's face—not angrily, but rather with "great patience and careful instruction." She felt she had already told him, but I encouraged that patient instruction meant telling him ten different times and in ten different ways: "Since retirement, your outside interests have pulled you away from me, and I miss regular lovemaking." Don't nag—lovingly confront your mate into needed changes.

Confrontation gets better with practice, but it's never fun or easy. God needs us to be the type of mate and companion who cares enough to wisely confront. Maturity can give us a deeper sense of commitment, a broader understanding of life, and less fear of being direct, which all augment this skill.

CONFESSING

James wrote, "Confess your trespasses to one another, and pray for one another, that you may be healed" (5:16 NKJV). "He who covers his sins will not prosper, but whoever confesses and forsakes them will have mercy" (Prov. 28:13 NKJV). Confession is crucial to healing intimate relationships that have been damaged by sinful behaviors, lazy neglect, or naive ignorance.

Confession includes two important processes:

1. *Bringing secrets to the light of day so we drain them of their power.* Satan loves to operate in secrecy and darkness. The secrets we refuse to admit will fester and gain greater destructiveness. If we bring them to the light of day, God gives us perspective. The person who confesses lusting after someone outside the marriage often finds the attraction greatly diminished the next time that person crosses his or her path.

2. *Confession also allows God and a caring person to see our ugliness and still love us.* We can begin to let go of guilt

and shame as we separate sin from sinner. We find out we are not impostors but redeemable sinners when a person knows all of our ugly secrets and *still* loves us.

An important part of this discipline is seeking out appropriate confessors that are trustworthy and wise. It's usually not healthy to make your wife or husband your only confessor. Men need a same-sex person to hear their confession and not overreact, bluntly tell it like it is, encourage, and hold their feet to the fire. Women need that female buddy to unload to and feel understood—and also to be exhorted toward growth.

REPENTING

Repentance is a frequent topic in the New Testament: "I hold this against you: You have forsaken your first love. Remember the height from which you have fallen! Repent and do the things you did at first" (Rev. 2:4–5 NIV). "Godly sorrow produces repentance leading to salvation, not to be regretted" (2 Cor. 7:10 NKJV). Repentance demonstrates that we recognize and accept responsibility for destructive thoughts and actions as we *choose to make necessary changes*. Repentance means giving feet to our remorse and making a 180-degree turn in the other direction. We are truly going to turn things around.

Wives so often say to me that their husbands become remorseful and make changes. The problem is that they usually last only about two months, and then they relapse into old attitudes and behaviors. Godly character change that results in sexual integrity is a process with many ongoing choices that will continue over a lifetime.

We must follow through on repentance and seek out all the destructive thinking and behaviors that are damaging our marriage and sex life and change them. Lovers can recapture their first love and move on to an intimacy they have never experienced before. Making changes and then *continuing* to make changes is the only way that a great marriage and love life can be built and flourish.

PUTTING EMOTIONS IN PERSPECTIVE

Emotions motivate and are given by God to be our servants. Some are short-term catalysts and can quickly sour if we hold on to them. These are God's tools for mending losses in those broken places, as He moves us back into places of joy and peace. Anger shows us justice has been violated. Guilt makes us aware of needed changes. Fear helps us to be protective, and jealousy can guard what is important. Envy shows us something is missing, while grief cleanses. Some emotions, like love, joy, contentment, and desire, are long-term, and we cultivate them for creating and nurturing intimacy.

In the ER, emotions are tuned in to and encouraged to do their servant function—but with cognitive guidance. The sooner we understand the purpose of the emotion, the quicker we can learn what we need to learn. Old age can be a boon and a detriment. Maturity can help us not hang on to false guilt but make necessary changes, and accept our situations without undue negative envy. Some feelings can also become bigger ghosts in later years because they have such a history, and aging has its many challenges that can trigger deep fears and anger. But God gives us the grace and wisdom to understand and manage even our most haunting feelings as we tune in to His bigger picture and gain perspective.

GRIEVING

"Blessed are those who mourn, for they shall be comforted" (Matt. 5:4 NKJV). "Rejoice with those who rejoice, and weep with those who weep" (Rom. 12:15 NKJV). Because we live in a broken world, we have to learn to cry. This grieving can take many forms, but all are filled with cleansing, healing tears as we work through those grieving stages of denial, anger, and hurt.

It is so comforting that God knew we would need to cry and heal our souls in this messy world. He promised that we "will be comforted." In older age grieving can be a complex process. A multitude of losses can confront us with parents in their eighties, aging bodies, and transitions into new lifestyles. These losses may be real or may be more abstract with a threatened or feared loss. Our grieving may also be cumulative, and the present loss may trigger grief over many past losses that have not been properly grieved and healed. Grieving is not a process that can be worked through totally alone. We need others to share the process with us. Hold each other and cry those comforting tears.

FORGIVING

Sexuality and intimacy are so full of mistakes, both sinful and immature, that we have to master forgiveness as one of God's healing arts. The psalmist describes our loving Father and His gently forgiving way as He compassionately operates in a fallen world: "The LORD is compassionate and gracious, slow to anger, abounding in love . . . he does not treat us as our sins deserve or repay us according to our iniquities . . . For he knows how we are formed, he remembers that we are dust [human]" (Ps. 103:8, 10, 14 NIV). The apostle Paul adds, "Therefore, as God's chosen people, holy and dearly loved, clothe yourselves with compassion, kindness, humility, gentleness and patience. *Bear with each other and forgive*" (Col. 3:12–13 NIV, emphasis added).

A genuine part of maturity is learning to live with all this ambiguity of human error and disappointed expectations. It is not by accident that Scripture encourages people to lovingly cut one another slack and learn to live the gentle, flexible life. The word *pardon* is an apt word for forgiveness. It is reconciling the ledger, even though justice has not been satisfied, as you keep a short account and quit blaming or resenting. We really aren't given an option on forgiving because God knew it was a necessity. We forgive because we are forgiven; we forgive in order to be forgiven. "Judge not . . . Condemn not . . . Forgive, and you will be forgiven" (Luke 6:37 NKJV).

The other person does not have to be repentant for us to forgive. We do it so we don't get eaten up with the cancer of resentment and revenge, thus blocking God's best for us. Remember that forgiveness is a process, and the most difficult person to forgive will often be yourself. Forgive your mate for his or her shortcomings, but of equal importance may be forgiving life and your aging body that lets you down at times. Maturity knows that a part of individually enjoying lovemaking is acceptance of present challenges and gently letting go of old realities to embrace new opportunities. It's about living forgiveness and flexibly opening up to new creative solutions.

BECOMING WHOLE

Two whole people create a whole marriage and a great sex life. Another function of God's emergency room is overcoming immaturity and skill deficits—growing up! Reading this book and finding other helpful teaching will go a long way in overcoming ignorance. One man came to counseling totally upset with his present sex life and the way his body was performing—with orgasms less powerful and his penis responding differently. He was afraid his sexuality was rapidly leaving him. What a relief as he discovered he was simply going through normal changes in aging and they were manageable. His sex life rapidly picked up after this counseling session.

Appropriating maturity is a lifelong process. More than knowledge, the paradigm shift of attitude and approach makes a whole lover. Learn these ER skills, especially grieving and forgiving. These skills aren't fun or easy, but we think you will find that your maturity will assist in attaining their mastery. They will help you build the passionately intimate marriage and sex life that you desire.

Chapter 20

Old Dogs Learn More Tricks:
Making Choices for Passionate Change

emember the formula for this final stage of the life span and how aging is not a choice—but our response is:

Changes bring **challenges**, which present us with **choices** that can lead to **creative solutions.**

As we have encouraged throughout the book, our attitudes and subsequent *choices* make the difference in whether our aging *challenges* fork into the high road (creative solutions) or the low road (negative existence). Our many transitions sexually bring complex challenges that motivate us into becoming great detectives to find creative solutions. This will be especially true of menopause, pesky arthritis, bouts of impotence, and many other things we have dealt with in this book.

How fascinating that in our mature years we can be content and whole, rather than rigid old fogies who bark at everybody and can't adapt. Mature people adapt more readily from a place of wisdom, not wanting to repeat mistakes. Old dogs indeed learn more tricks because we desire and can more easily achieve a deeper quality of life.

As you ponder the joys of growing older, remember that *maturity is not a given with age*. Everyone ages, but becoming mature is an individual process that involves many choices and much growing up. All of us know immature sixty-year-olds in whom the lessons of life haven't created wisdom. Pondering what it means to grow wise and not just grow old brings some fascinating issues to the table. In this concluding chapter, let's consider some of the characteristics of mature people.

SEVEN TRAITS OF THE TRULY MATURE PERSON

Here are seven traits we think must be cultivated to bring about the paradigm shift into new concepts for enjoying these mature years. Maturity can be the catalyst for a deeper sexual intimacy and a greater enjoyment of lovemaking.

1. Maturity lives gracefully with ambiguity, mess, mistakes, and humanness. Maturity accepts, forgives, and moves on more easily and graciously. Have any of our lives turned out the way we planned? I doubt it. In youth, life can be black and white without shades of gray. This world is sinful and fallen, and we are fallible humans. Maturity graciously accepts others, forgives, and cuts people slack. Perfection need not be achieved for comfortable compromise and joyful living.

As we accept the complexities of life, we discover that this place of dissonance and confusion is used by God to launch us into some marvelous blessings and solutions. Control is an illusion. Accepting uncertainty and the possibility of mistakes is the initial step into growth. Old age tolerantly moves through the mess to claim joys and victories. As that famous philosopher Jimmy Buffett states, "Some of it's magic, some of it's tragic, but I had a good life all the way."

Sexual intimacy is full of difficulty and humanness. Maturity allows a husband to make love joyously to his wife who has had a mastectomy or is working through a terrible menopause. Orgasms may not feel like a volcano, but the excitement can still flood our bodies and relationships. Shifts and choices keep the warmth and passion present in new and deeper ways. It doesn't have to be perfect, but it can be comfortable and tenderly connecting.

2. *Maturity postpones immediate pleasure for long-term gain.* An adolescent in tenth grade has a difficult time understanding that a failed math test could impact a semester's grade and in turn his choice of colleges. The Saturday dance seems all important, but maturity knows the importance of delayed gratification. As the old preacher Bob Jones used to emphasize, "Never sacrifice the permanent on the altar of the immediate."

There is more to life than just today, and perspective

quiets the drama. Old age can more easily distinguish between a 2 and a 10 in order of importance. Some hills aren't worth dying on. Maturity is less reactive to the temporary and works to achieve long-term goals.

We keep our precious grandbaby most every Wednesday night. I [Doug] was looking forward to enjoying some intimate time together this past Thursday morning before Caitlyn woke up—only to be interrupted by cries of, "Papa, Papa, come get me." We thought those days of postponement were over. These and other delayed gratifications come easier, especially if they promote needed intimacy. Maturity allows us to foresee that helping a mate through a health crisis may take precedence over personal gratification—only to discover new levels of passion.

3. Maturity knows how to suffer graciously and embrace reality (the rules)—especially our own mortality. Accepting losses then grieving and moving through them becomes an accepted and expected way of life, which opens the door to new opportunities. Christians can somehow get into a mind-set that says suffering means God has withdrawn His blessing. Jesus knew that this is a broken world and actually God draws His children closer through suffering. He emphasized, "Blessed are those who mourn, for they will be comforted" (Matt. 5:4 NIV). The changes of aging, especially sexual, can incorporate some losses. Again, these challenges also bring choices for new depths of sexual intimacy.

Youth believes they are ten feet tall and bulletproof—natural consequences can be avoided. Maturity knows the rules apply—we're born, we live, we die. Accepting mortality creates a profound understanding of the circle of life. This can motivate us to finish strong and more deeply enjoy each moment of the final years, not losing valuable time to fear, envy, and regret.

Sexual intimacy in aging accepts losses and learns how to play through the physical disabilities. We don't have to keep a happy face but can cry over losing our favorite position of intercourse to arthritis. In our later years, sex may occur without orgasms, and loving looks and touch may take precedence over intercourse.

4. *Maturity understands the importance of intimacy and creating a quality of life. Maturity sees life and success as a process—not a goal.* You know that old story of having never heard a person on their deathbed wishing they could have spent more time at work. With age and wisdom comes a shifting of priorities and values. Being with your mate, relaxing with friends, spending time with the grandchildren, and playing golf with buddies take on new significance.

The busyness of life and surviving take precedence in younger years. This hectic pace detracts from quality of life and availability to intimacy. Maturity starts to achieve balance. Relationships become more important than accruing more assets, and achievements are measured on God's scales as to what lives we have touched. It's a different measuring stick of success and where to sink energy.

Vacationing creates many natural aphrodisiacs. Holding hands and much time spent together with fewer interruptions, an anticipation of intimate times—all these can be a part of older empty-nest companionship. Creating a priority for sharing lives and enjoying long-awaited dreams bring couples closer together.

5. Maturity builds wonderfully rich sexual intimacy. We mentioned earlier that a case could be made that intimate lovemaking is wasted on those less than fifty years of age. Scripture uses the word *know* for sexual lovemaking. Maturity has the kind of accepting and understanding wisdom necessary to truly know a mate. This will be much more likely to occur at fifty than at thirty.

6. Maturity has incorporated God's gift of self-esteem with a true servant's heart. Scripture encourages servanthood—that ability to reach out beyond our own desires to meet the needs of another. We are asked to submit ourselves one to another. This loving humility is based on a maturity of being comfortable in our own skin and acknowledging God's verdict that each of us is uniquely and wonderfully made (see Ps. 139:14). From that strong place of self-acceptance, we have nothing to prove.

Sexual intimacy flourishes when two psychologically whole people can relax in their own bodies and revel in their sexual feelings. Each lover can comfortably nurture the other and enjoy creating sexual arousal and fulfillment in their partner. Mature lovers are comfortable in their own skin and tenderly meet one another's needs.

7. Maturity recognizes the importance of faith and God's loving, wise perspective. Aging brings us closer to heaven and eternity. Jesus, redemption, and an eternal perspective give us the ability to face our mortality and death with a peace that conquers the unknown. Aging brings with it much uncharted territory and unpredictable challenges. God promises to be there with comfort and purpose, and we learn wonderful ways to crawl up into the lap of the Almighty: "He who dwells in the shelter

of the Most High will rest in the shadow of the Almighty"
(Ps. 91:1 NIV).

God's love and eternal purpose grow sweeter with
maturity. His wisdom can permeate our lives in wonderful ways that make us enjoy relationships even more.
Grandparenting, friendships, and mentoring take on
whole new meanings. Drawing nearer to God brings us
closer to each other.

We hope you will work to become increasingly more
mature—not just older. These are marvelous years of
sexual celebration and deep intimacy. We know that just
reading a book is never enough. I [Doug] come from a
Baptist background, and we always had altar calls at the
end of presentations. This was a time of coming forward
and making decisions and changes around what we had
just heard. Let us make an altar call with some final suggestions for applying this book.

Affirming your choices for a loving companionship
and greater sexual intimacy:

1. Keep a log of time spent together as a couple—how
could you increase this in the coming months?

2. Go over old pictures and memories and affirm your
history and traditions.

3. As you have read this book, which area of your
marital intimacy have you discovered is the strongest,
and which needs the most changes?

4. If your mate would read and apply only one chapter in the book—which one would you choose? Which
one would they choose for you?

5. Think through the chapter your mate chose for you and the areas needing the most changes. Pick three challenges that you choose to change into more positive solutions.

May God give you the wisdom and courage during this wonderful time of life to create a true celebration of sex. Remember to keep making those choices!

Changes bring **challenges**, which present us with **choices** that can lead to **creative solutions.**

Notes and Resources

CHAPTER 3

1. This information comes from the North American Menopause Society Web site at www.menopause.org.
2. L. Dennerstein, A. Smith, C. Morse, and H. Burger, "Sexuality and Menopause," *Journal of Psychosomatic Obstetrics & Gynecology* 15 (1994): 59–66.
3. C. Penner and J. Penner, "Senior Sex," *Christian Counseling Today* 7 (1999): 13–16.
4. Ibid.
5. G. Trudel, L. Turgeon, and L. Piche, "Marital and Sexual Aspects of Old Age," *Sexual and Relationship Therapy* 15(4) (2000): 385.
6. Ibid.
7. B. Rienzo, "The Impact of Aging on Human Sexuality," *Journal of School Health* 55 (1985): 66–68.
8. L. Fazio, "Sexuality and Aging: A Community Wellness Program," *Physical and Occupational Therapy in Geriatrics* 6 (1987): 59–69.

CHAPTER 4

1. L. Dennerstein, E. Dudley, et al., "A Prospective Population-Based Study of Menopausal Symptoms," *Obstetrics and Gynecology* 96 (2000): 351–57.
2. C. Penner and J. Penner, "Senior Sex."
3. C. Meston and P. Frohlich, "The Neurobiology of Sexual Function," *Archives of General Psychiatry* 57 (2000): 1012–30.
4. T. Crenshaw and J. Goldberg, *Sexual Pharmacology: Drugs That Affect Sexual Functioning* (New York: W. W. Norton & Co, 1996).
5. This information comes from the Health Scout on-line newsletter, which can be accessed at www.healthscout.com.
6. T. Crenshaw and J. Goldberg, *Sexual Pharmacology*.
7. This information comes from the Women's Health Interactive *Midlife Health Center* Web site: www.womens-health.com.
8. This information was taken from an Associated Press article

posted on the PsyUSA listserve entitled "Antidepressants Used to Ease Hot Flashes," December 29, 2003.

9. M. Mayo and J. Mayo, *The Menopause Manager* (Grand Rapids: Fleming Revell, 1998).

10. Meston and Frohlich, "The Neurobiology of Sexual Function."

11. W. Yates, "Testosterone and Behavior," *Essential Psychopharmacology* 4(4) (2002): 261–78.

The following Web sites are also useful resources:

North American Menopause Society, P.O. Box 94527, Cleveland, OH 44101-4527, ph. 440-442-7550, www.menopause.org

American College of Obstetrics and Gynecology, Office of Public Information, 409 12th St. NW, Washington, DC 20024-2188, ph. 202-638-5577, www.acog.org.

Menopause-Online provides up-to-date information and offers overviews of signs symptoms, and traditional and alternative treatments. www.menopause-online.com

Power Surge is a virtual community for women in the pause. There are medical/expert recommendations, members sharing experiences, and a comprehensive hyperlinked index of menopause related resources. www.dearest.com

OBGYN.net – Menopause is a physician-reviewed service offering medical information and interaction on menopause. www.obgynet/women/conditions/hc-menopause.htm

CHAPTER 5

1. B. Bass, "The Medicalization of Male Sexuality," *Maryland Psychologist* 48(3) (2003): 11, 17.

2. T. Crenshaw and J. Goldberg, *Sexual Pharmacology.*

3. Ibid.

4. Ibid.

5. S. Lamberts, A. Van den Beld, and A. van der Lely, "The Endocrinology of Aging," *Science* 278 (1997): 419–24.

CHAPTER 6

1. A. Hart, C. Hart Webber, and D. Taylor, *Secrets of Eve: Understanding the Mystery of Female Sexuality* (Nashville: Word, 1998).

2. N. Fairbanks, *Death a l'Orange* (New York: Berkley, 2002).

3. S. Davidson, "Hot! Hot! Hot!," *Reader's Digest*, August (2003), 75.

CHAPTER 7

1. J. Block, *Sex Over 50* (West Nyack, N.Y.: Parker, 1999).
2. T. LaHaye and B. LaHaye, *The Act of Marriage after 40* (Grand Rapids, MI: Zondervan, 2000).

CHAPTER 8

1. E. Boyce and E. Umland, "Sildenafil Citrate: A Therapeutic Update," *Clinical Therapy* 23(1) (2001): 2–23.
2. R. Rosen, "Erectile Dysfunction in Middle-Aged and Older Men," *Handbook of Clinical Sexuality for Mental Health Professionals*, S. Levine, ed. (New York: Brunner-Routledge, 2003), 240–44.
3. This information came from a workshop by Mary Gutierrez, Pharm.D., entitled "Good sexual function and what can go wrong."
4. The chapter "Women Becoming More Easily Orgasmic" in *A Celebration of Sex* by Douglas Rosenau (Nashville: Thomas Nelson, 2002) is a very helpful resource to address orgasmic difficulties.

The following Web sites are also useful resources:

WebMD has an Impotence Health Center with information regarding the up-to-date research in the area of sexual dysfunction: www.webmd.com.

Also, Medscape from WebMD has an Erectile Dysfunction Resource Center with articles regarding research and medication information: www.medscape.com.

The American Urological Association provides comprehensive patient information regarding disorders and treatments: www.auanet.org.

The American Urological Association also has an on-line patient information resource that was written by urology experts and is accompanied by medical illustrations when appropriate: www.urologyhealth.org.

The Sexual Function Health Council of the American Foundation for Urologic Diseases, Inc., has sponsored this site: www.impotence.org.

The Vulvar Pain Foundation provides information on sexual pain disorders (e.g., vestibulitis, vulvodynia, dyspareunia): www.vulvarpainfoundation.org.

On the Senior Living Web site you can find resources for those looking for information on sex after fifty: www.seniorliving.about.com/cs/sexafter50.

CHAPTER 9

1. J. Block, *Sex Over 50*.
2. American Heart Association, *Sex and Heart Disease* [Brochure] (Dallas, TX: 2001).
3. This information was taken from an article on the American Cancer Society Web site, "Sexuality for Men and Their Partners," (2003): www.cancer.org.
4. American Heart Association, *Together Again: Our Guide to Intimacy After Stroke* [Brochure] (Dallas, TX: 2001).

The following Web sites are also useful resources:

American Cancer Society; www.cancer.org; ph. 1-800-ACS-2345; or call your local American Cancer Society for information on cancer, its treatment, and sexuality.

American Diabetes Association; www.diabetes.com; ph. 1-800-DIABETES; 1701 North Beauregard Street, Alexandria, VA 22311.

American Heart Association; www.americanheart.org; ph. 1-800-242-8721; 7272 Greenville Avenue, Dallas, TX 75231-4596. Information on heart disease, stroke, and sexuality.

Arthritis Foundation; www.arthritis.org; ph. 1-800-283-7800; P.O. Box 7669, Atlanta, GA 30357-0669. Information on arthritis and sexuality.

CHAPTER 10

1. A. Riley, M. Peet, C. Wilson, eds., *Sexual Pharmacology* (New York: Oxford University Press, 1993).
2. T. Crenshaw and J. Goldberg, *Sexual Pharmacology*.
3. Ibid.
4. R. Virag, P. Bouilly, and D. Frydman, "Is Impotence an Arterial Disorder?" *Lancet* 1 (1985): 181.
5. T. Crenshaw and J. Goldberg, *Sexual Pharmacology*. Much of the medication information in this chapter is summarized from this Crenshaw and Goldberg text.
6. B. Boyarsky and R. Hirschfeld, "The Management of Medication-Induced Sexual Dysfunction," *Essential Psychopharmacology* 3(2) (2000): 39–58.
7. Ibid.

8. A. Cohen, *Ginkgo Biloba for Drug-Induced Sexual Dysfunction,* 1997 American Psychiatric Association meetings, San Diego, CA.
9. C. Meston and P. Frohlich, "The Neurobiology of Sexual Function."

CHAPTER 11

1. This information was taken from a Reuters Health on-line article entitled "Pfizer Says Viagra May Work as Fast as Rivals," December 2002.
2. J. Block, *Sex Over 50.*
3. K. Peterson, "Till Viagra Do Us Part? Side Effects: A Factor in Affairs and Divorces as Drug Moves into Mainstream Use," *USA Today,* March 22, 2001.
4. M. Scott Peck, *The Road Less Traveled* (New York: Simon & Schuster, 1978).

CHAPTER 12

1. For a more complete discussion on this topic, we recommend the chapter "Sexual Desire and Frequency" (with Michael Sytsma and Debra Taylor) in *A Celebration of Sex* by Douglas Rosenau (Nashville: Thomas Nelson, 2002).
2. A. Hart, C. Hart Webber, and D. Taylor, *Secrets of Eve.*
3. W. Backus and M. Chapian, *Telling Yourself the Truth* (Minneapolis: Bethany House, 1980).
4. A. Hart, C. Hart Webber, and D. Taylor, *Secrets of Eve.*
5. T. Crenshaw and J. Goldberg, *Sexual Pharmacology.*

CHAPTER 14

1. Christopher McCluskey and his wife, Rachel, have a fascinating book on the Lovemaking Cycle with Baker/Revell Publishers: *When Two Become One.* He also has an excellent videotape, "Coaching Couples into Passionate Intimacy," which explains the model and can be ordered through his Web site: www.christian-living.com.

CHAPTER 15

1. A. Hart, C. Hart Webber, and D. Taylor, *Secrets of Eve.*

Index

Acknowledgments

Catherine Rosenau supported us through some grueling writing weekends with food, encouragement and making sure we took breaks. She is indeed the wind beneath Doug's wings and has our heartfelt gratitude for her many contributions.

Jim and Carolyn are grateful to Coleman, Chanda, Sara, Jeff, and Scott, who put up with their parents in this process and are such a blessing to our home.

Carolyn expresses appreciation to her Women's Bible Study who had the courage to share their experiences and their prayers; to Dale Philp and Sue Allinson who laughed and cried with her; and to her "Daddy" whose love was unconditional, whose prayers were life changing, and who she misses so much.

With a special bond and deep appreciation, we thank our baby boomer friends and sex therapy colleagues: Sue Townsend, Debbie Neel, Ellen Fox, Vickie George, Phil Drake, Lauren Spooner, and Sandy Myers. As the "Maturity Rocks!" gang, you gave such great suggestions and editing help for this book.

A hearty thanks goes to Christopher McCluskey who allowed the inclusion of his Lovemaking Cycle and to his colleagues in the organization Sexual Wholeness, Michael Sytsma and Debra Taylor, who helped create the chapter on desire and did valuable editing.

We would also like to thank Dr. Stephen Lippman and

Dr. Mitesh Kothari, an endocrinologist and OB-GYN who've helped make this journey easier; Dr. Gary Oliver, Dr. Howard Eyrich, and Dr. Bill Hines, colleagues and teachers who believed and encouraged.

We appreciate Alan Tiegreen for creating the illustrations for the book.

Thank you, Thomas Nelson, for making this book possible. Your motivation and skilled assistance, especially Pete Nikolai and our editors, Beth Ann Patton and Elizabeth Kea, helped create this needed addition to the baby boomer library.

About the Authors

Dr. Douglas R. Rosenau is a licensed psychologist, marriage and family therapist, and diplomate of the American Board of Sexology. Cofounder of the Christian organization, Sexual Wholeness, Dr. Rosenau is an adjunct professor at Reformed Theological Seminary and Psychological Studies Institute. He lives in Atlanta with his wife, Cathy; they have one daughter and one grandchild.

Dr. James K. Childerston is a clinical psychologist specializing in problems associated with anxiety, depression, sexual abuse, male sexuality, and marital concerns. He serves as the vice president of the Academy of Medical Psychology and is on the national advisory board of the Christian Care Network (CCN). He is the coauthor of *Purity & Passion: Authentic Male Sexuality*. He and his wife, Carolyn, and five children reside in Hagerstown, Maryland.

Carolyn Sue Childerston is the Practice Administrator for Childerston and Associates, a psychological private practice in Hagerstown, Maryland. She regularly consults with women regarding hormone-related concerns and is an author and speaker in this specialty area. Carolyn has an M.A. in Biblical Counseling from Trinity College and Seminary.